from Medical Center
Houston, on Main
Holiday Inn Medical

ASTHMA

PRACTICAL CLINICAL MEDICINE

Series Editors J. Fry and G. Sandler

ASTHMA

Edited by G. Jariwalla

Consultant Physician
Bromley and Tunbridge Wells
Health Authorities

MTP PRESS LIMITED
a member of the KLUWER ACADEMIC PUBLISHERS GROUP
LANCASTER / BOSTON / THE HAGUE / DORDRECHT

Published in the UK and Europe by
MTP Press Limited
Falcon House
Lancaster, England

British Library Cataloguing in Publication Data

Asthma.
1. Man. Bronchi. Asthma
I. Jariwalla, G. (Gulamabbas) II. Series
616.2′38

ISBN 0–85200–672–1
ISBN 0–85200–821–X Series

Published in the USA by
MTP Press
A division of Kluwer Academic Publishers
101 Philip Drive
Norwell, MA 02061, USA

Typeset, printed and bound in Great Britain by
Butler & Tanner Ltd, Frome and London

Contents

Authors

Dr G. Jariwalla, MB, BCh (Wales), MRCP (UK)
Consultant Physician,
Bromley and Tunbridge Wells Health Authorities

Dr J.P.R. Hartley, MD, MRCP
Consultant Physician,
Brighton Health District

Dr P.J. Rees, MD, MRCP
Consultant Physician, and Senior Lecturer
Guy's Hospital, London

Dr J.B. Macdonald, MD, FRCP
Consultant Physician,
Ayrshire and Arran Health Board

Dr E.H.Walters, MD, MRCP
Consultant Physician,
Newcastle General Hospital
Newcastle-upon-Tyne

Series Editors' Foreword

Backing up the pioneering medical researchers and experimenters are the phalanxes and cohorts of practising clinicians in district general hospitals and in general practice who may have to implement and apply any breakthroughs and advances in practical and realistic terms. This they cannot, and should not, be expected to do without careful consideration and analysis. It is essential, therefore, to have regular reviews of the growing points of medicine which are constructively critical as well as being enthusiastic and which can present the issues and implications clearly and fairly to clinicians.

The *Practical Clinical Medicine* series is designed to provide such regular reviews on selected subjects. Each volume is under the charge of an invited editor who selects his team of 4–6 experts. Each contribution is an authoritative, detailed and referenced examination of his topic, is clearly presented in an understandable manner and is practical, relevant and applicable to everyday clinical practice.

The series is intended as a means of communication between researchers and practising clinicians. It is dedicated to generalists who provide primary health care in general practice and to generalists providing secondary medical care in district general hospitals. Both are involved in applying good general practical clinical medicine for their patients, but can only succeed in a climate of constant review and examination.

JOHN FRY
GERALD SANDLER

1

INTRODUCTION

Asthma is a common complaint,[1] whether one looks at the paediatric or adult population. It is estimated that 10% of the population could be labelled 'asthmatics' at some stage especially if wheezing and cough are regarded as the main

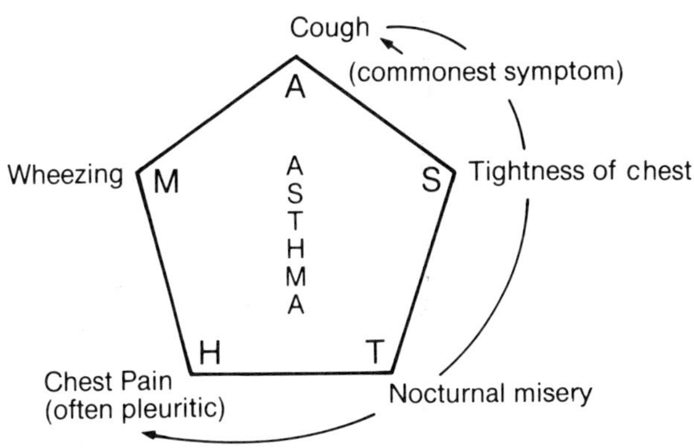

Figure 1.1 Symptoms of asthma

recurrent symptoms (Fig. 1.1). Any two of the symptoms shown in Fig. 1.1 should make a doctor strongly suspicious of the diagnosis – more than two of these would confirm the presence of asthma.

Should the definition of asthma be clinical or pathological?

Ideally it should contain both aspects, i.e. a condition characterized by episodes of breathlessness with wheeze and cough which responds well to treatment – the bronchospasm due to bronchial hypersensitivity and production of thick viscid sputum. Opinions vary among doctors and research scientists on the patho-physiology and management of this potentially disabling and severe disease and in Chapters 3 and 4 we discuss critically and in detail current views on these aspects.

Do the majority of childhood asthmatics spontaneously recover and subsequently go into remission? Many parents ask this question. Asthma is an unpredictable disorder and should be 'sold' to the patient and relative as such. However, there is good statistical evidence that the majority of children will 'grow out' of this condition in their late teens. Martin *et al.*[2] followed over 300 children from the age of seven years until 21 years old, by which time 55% were wheeze-free. There was an improvement in 75% of those who constantly wheezed between seven years of age and adolescence by the time they reached 21 years of age. This phenomenon is obviously in many ways a reversal of adult asthma – why? One possible explanation is the effect of 'growth' on airway structure since a doubling of airways can result in a 16-fold reduction in airway resistance.

Is asthma underdiagnosed? Lee *et al.*[3] asked over 2500 seven-year-old children whether they had wheezed over the previous two years. They found positive answers in 11%, whereas the recognized prevalence of asthma in children varies between 1.8–4.2%. When 1300 children were given histamine provocation, 60% of wheezing children had PC_{20} histamine levels of less than 16 mg/ml which correlated with the severity of their asthma. Of the 'normal' children (who had not wheezed), 30% had PC_{20} histamine levels of less than 16 mg/ml. In contrast, of 2000 adults 23% had wheezed within the previous 2 years. The recognized prevalence of asthma in adults is 4% but when these adults were investigated with respect to PC_{20} values no association was found between wheeze and shortness of breath. It is well recognized that if young asthmatics less than

Aggravating and precipitating factors

- Majority of asthma is 'cryptogenic'
- Infections – bacterial
  – viral
  – miscellaneous
- Allergic influences
- Occupational (isocyanates)
- Drugs (NSAIDs)
- Exercise
- Psychological factors
- Pregnancy
- Menstrual

21 years of age could be treated properly then the permanent, severe asthmatic state may not develop.

The mast cell and the mediators it releases is crucial in producing bronchoconstriction (Fig. 1.2). Should there be a rationalized form of management in asthma or individual choices? This question can only be answered if different methods of treatment are compared in terms of efficacy and cost. Such studies are not available. The aims of treatment should be to achieve as normal lung function as possible, maintain good quality of life and make the drug regime 'simple' to follow. The hope of every asthmatic is for a cure. However, recognizing the unpredictability of this condition, it would be wise not to prognosticate but to offer effective management (see Fig. 1.3).

Allergy influences are complex and conflicting. For allergy tests (including RAST) to be meaningful, a detailed history from the patient is essential. Skin (prick) testing on the whole is reliable, easy and safe. Nasal provocation testing, however, is risky and should be carried out only at 'specialist' centres. Positive reactions to prick tests in conjunction with blood

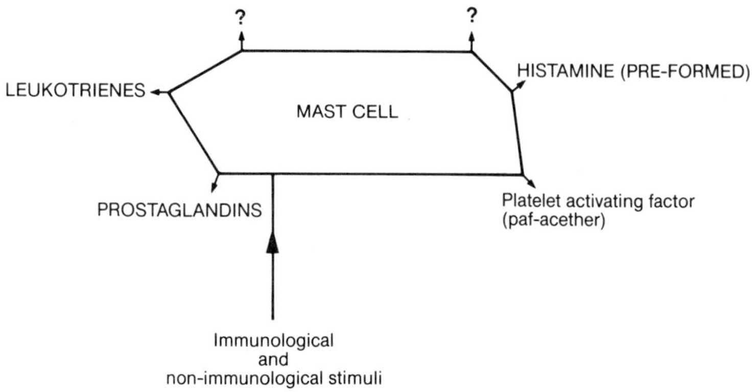

Figure 1.2 Role of mast cell in bronchoconstriction

Aims of treatment

- Lung function
  FEV_1 FVC–80–90%
  Lung volumes normal
  PEFR ~ 80% predicted
- Quality of life
  No restriction in occupation and activities (social & athletic)
  Minimal or no time lost off work
- Drug regime
  Inhaled in most cases
  Twice daily if possible

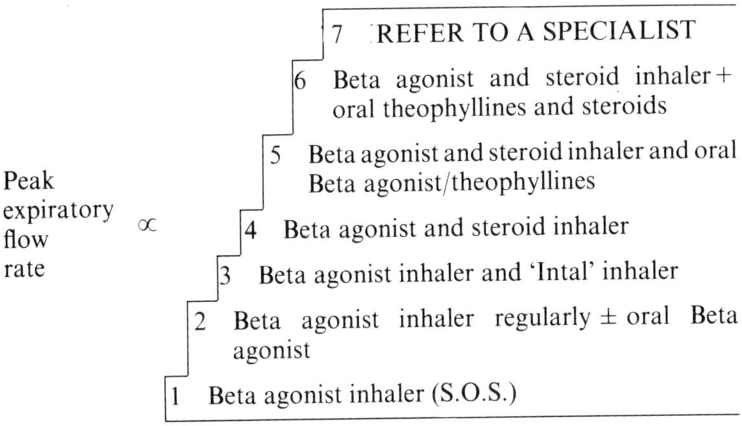

Figure 1.3 Broad 'types' of treatment featured in an escalator fashion. From Paterson & Tarata (1981)[4]

eosinophilia, and finding of eosinophils, Curschmann's spirals and Charcot–Leyden crystals would favour a diagnosis of extrinsic asthma. Elevated total IgE levels are found in this group of asthmatics. Three logical steps in the treatment of an allergic patient are:

(1) Avoidance or elimination of the allergies.
(2) Symptomatic – using drugs, e.g. steroids, cromoglycate, antihistamines.
(3) Immunotherapy using allergen extracts – either the shorter course of alum-precipitated slow-release material or a longer aqueous type of mixture.

Medical interest in occupational aspects of asthma dates as far back as the sixteenth century with observations by Agricola and Paracelsus. A history from an asthmatic patient is incomplete if it does not contain details of his occupation. Over 200 substances – dusts, vapours and fumes – are implicated in the production of occupational asthma. The incidence of occupational asthma varies according to the 'type' and quantity of exposure and overall is estimated to affect 20% of workers. A significant proportion of employees in, for example, the electronic industry, were supposed to have left because of respiratory disease[5].

The three main groups of occupational asthma sufferers are bakers, housewives, e.g. using 'biological' soap powders and those working in the pharmaceutical industry. Atopic individuals become more readily sensitized to the enzymes of Bacillus subtilis used in 'biological' soap-powders than non-atopic workers. However, in toluene-di-isocyanate (TDI) related asthma there appears to be no relationship between the atopic and non-atopic state. Prevention of these occupationally-related diseases should be the main aim of the doctor. It may be advisable to exclude atopic workers from occupations in which there is a high risk from exposure to certain allergens, bakery, detergent industry and metal-refining industry. This can only be achieved at the pre-employment stage when those with family or previous history of allergy are identified. The United States Bureau of Labour (1956) listed over 100 occupations related to asthma whilst in France in 1960, the first occupational asthma to be recognized was that associated with handling penicillin. In the UK, occupational asthma resulting from a restricted list of sensitizing agents has now been accepted as a prescribed industrial disease[6].

Purely psychological stimuli may contribute towards the production of 'asthma'. This is demonstrated by a story which Trousseau, himself an asthmatic, tells in his *Lectures on Clinical Medicine*: 'The worst fit of asthma which I ever had myself came on under the following circumstance. I suspected my coachman of dishonesty, and in order to assure myself of this I went upstairs to the loft one day and had the oats measured in my presence, whilst this was being done I was all at once seized with a fit of dyspnoea and oppression of the chest so great that I had scarcely the strength to get back to my apartment, my eyeballs protruded out of their sockets and my pale and turgid face expressed the deepest anxiety. I had only time to pull my tie off and to rush to the window, which I opened in search of fresh air. I am not a habitual smoker but

I then had a cigar and took a few puffs; in eight or ten minutes the paroxysm was over. What had caused this fit? Doubtless it was the dust from the oats which were being measured that penetrated into my bronchi. But it was unquestionable also that this dust was not enough to bring on of itself such an extraordinary attack or the cause at least was quite out of proportion to the effect produced. I have a hundred times in the streets, or on the boulevards of Paris or on the high roads, been exposed to an atmosphere of dust considerably thicker than the one which I had breathed for a very short time, and yet I had never felt anything approaching this. There must, therefore, have been something special in the cause, and it had besides acted on me whilst I was in a peculiar state. My nervous system was shaken from the influence of mental emotion caused by the idea of a theft, however trifling, committed by one of my servants, and a cause, very slight in itself, had acted on my nerves with extreme intensity.' The above account demonstrates very well the multiplicity of influences in asthma: physical, constitutional, allergic and psychological.

There is a fairly general idea that a high proportion of asthmatics are to be found amongst the more intelligent sections of the community. There may be some truth in this but this is not to say that less intelligent groups do not have asthma. As a group, asthmatics tend to be self-assertive and possibly slightly more aggressive and emotionally less stable. From the earliest work on asthma (Sir John Floyer in 1698) to the present day, the hereditary influences are well emphasized. The family history may be of asthma, urticaria, hay fever, rhinitis, eczema or migraine.

Unger stated in 1944: 'In comparison with other chronic diseases such as chronic arthritis and cardiovascular renal disease, the results of treatment in asthma are usually brilliant. In those who do not obtain complete relief there is usually amelioration of symptoms, i.e. the attacks of asthma are milder and less frequent. Failures occur of course but in only a small minority and are often due to negligence on the part of the patient (or parent) or of the physician.' Similarly, Urbach and Gottlieb stated in *Allergy* (1946) 'The great majority of physicians are of the opinion that asthma is a dangerous but practically an incurable disease. Although they naturally refrain from expressing this opinion to the patient, the latter very soon senses this pessimistic attitude which very often does immeasurable harm psychologically and consequently physically. The physician who is convinced that many cases can be cured and that almost all can be considerably improved and who is able to communicate this conviction to his patient, possesses the most important pre-requisite for success.'

Management of asthma includes social and psycho-social aspects in many patients; therefore family doctors (GPs) should really manage most of the individuals. In reality the trend is increasingly taking away management from the practice to hospitals, often to general physicians who may not have a special interest in respiratory medicine, let alone asthma. Is this move to be lamented? Anderson *et al.*[7] found, during an 8 year period in the South-West Thames Region, a five-fold increase in the number of children referred to hospital for the management of acute asthma without the previous intervention by their family doctors. This trend can not be explained in terms of the 'direct' referral system operated by many hospitals. A family doctor needs to earn the respect of an asthmatic patient, especially the child and his family unit if this trend of direct admissions is to be reversed. However, protagonists of the direct admission policy would quote a recent enquiry which concluded that it has probably succeeded in saving lives[8]. We believe that so long as doubt exists in a general practitioner's ability to recognize a 'severe' attack and the lack of wider use of peak flow meters and corticosteroids, there will be reasons to believe that 'dual' care, with hospitals taking the 'major' share, is fully justified[9].

When asthmatic patients are referred to specialists the general practitioner should state his willingness to accept responsibility to continue management on the recommended lines, otherwise the majority of the patients will remain with the specialist. After their first visit to the hospital when they are likely to see the 'specialist', subsequent assessment would often be undertaken by 'juniors' who may make no changes in the management and often will be less experienced than the family doctor. Chapter 6 includes examples of referral letters and discusses in each case:

(1) whether the diagnosis of asthma was made;
(2) if made or suggested was it the right one;
(3) treatment already offered;
(4) problems in the management;
(5) why treatment failed;
(6) what lines did the specialist pursue; and
(7) the outcome.

REFERENCES

1. Clarke T.J.H. and Godfrey S. (eds.) (1982). *Epidemiology in Asthma* (London: Chapman & Hall)
2. Martin A.J., McLennon L.A., Landau L.I. and Phelan P.D. (1980). The natural history of childhood asthma to adult life. *Br. Med. J.,* **280**, 1397–1400
3. Lee D.A., Winslow N.R., Speight A.N. and Hey E.N. (1983). Prevalence of asthma in childhood. *Br. Med. J.,* **286**, 1256–8
4. Paterson J.W. and Tarata R.A. (1981). Asthma; common pitfalls in management. *New Ethicals*, **18**, 39–51
5. Perks W.H., Burge, P.S., Rehahn M. and Green M. (1979). Work related respiratory disease in employees leaving an electronic factory. *Thorax*, **34**, 19
6. Department of Health and Social Security. (1981). *Occupational asthma – report by Industrial Injuries Advisory Council.* London: HMSO
7. Anderson H.A., Bailey P. and West S. (1979). Trends in the hospital care of acute childhood asthma 1970–78. A regional study. *Br. Med. J.*, **281**, 1190–4
8. Crompton G.K., Grant I.W.B. and Bloomfield P. (1979). Edinburgh emergency asthma admission service; report on 10 years experience. *Br. Med. J.*, **2**, 1199–1201
9. Arnold A.G., Lane D.J. amd Zapata E. (1983). Acute severe asthma; factors that influence hospital referral by general practitioner and self-referral by the patient. *Br. J. Dis. Chest*, **77**, 51–9

2

EPIDEMIOLOGY OF ASTHMA AND ASTHMA DEATHS

WHY BOTHER WITH EPIDEMIOLOGY?

Epidemiology is the study of factors influencing the frequency and distribution of a disease. Only epidemiology can tell us whether asthma is increasing or declining as a disease. Epidemiology can also assess the natural history of asthma, with its highly variable age of onset and disease profile. Only in this way can we get an all-round picture of the problem that asthma presents. Prevalence surveys in different communities show substantial differences. Changes in associated factors could shed light on more fundamental aspects of asthma aetiology. Genetic and migrant studies can explore the roles of heredity and environment in the disease. These insights are normally not available by any other technique, so asthma epidemiology could well be important.

Epidemiology can give valuable insights into asthma

Nonetheless, the epidemiology of asthma is beset by two major problems – the problem of defining asthma and the variety of survey methods used.

DEFINING ASTHMA

No one can survey a disease unless they can define it accurately. However, asthma is virtually impossible to define exactly. The broad consensus definition is 'a disease characterized by wide variations over short periods of time in resistance to flow in intrapulmonary airways[1]. Obviously this definition leaves many questions unanswered. What is a 'wide' variation? Is wheezing associated with chronic bronchitis included? A major problem is that every person has some degree of airways resistance variation according to time of day, temperature of inhaled air, etc. There appears to be a continuous spectrum between normal variation and asthma, with no clear cut-off point.

A central feature of asthma is agreed to be bronchial hyper-reactivity. Asthmatics have a greater degree of bronchoconstriction than normals in response to a challenge such as inhaled aerosol histamine or methacholine. Unfortunately, bronchial hyper-reactivity also appears to be a continuum with normals and asthmatics as the two extremes[2]. Subjects with intermediate degrees of reactivity are not uncommon. Thus defining asthma by bronchial hyper-reactivity is no easier than by variation of air flow resistance.

Diagnostic criteria for asthma that are too strict will result in missed cases but criteria that are too liberal will lead to the false inclusion of several other diseases. Wheezing can occur with chronic bronchitis and often responds to bronchodilator drugs. No current definitions of asthma exclude this category. So here is a grey area between asthma and chronic bronchitis. The perceived relationship between 'wheezy bronchitis' and asthma in children is slowly changing. In the past these were considered to be separate diseases, but this differentiation is being increasingly questioned. Studies in Melbourne[3] and Tyneside[4] have shown that these two conditions cannot be separated epidemiologically. Wheezy bronchitis and asthma are increasingly seen as symptoms of a common basic disorder[9].

> Wheezy bronchitis and asthma are essentially the same disease

Defining asthma objectively

Ideally one would be able to define whether or not every individual in a survey has asthma by a simple, reproducible, safe test. But we are a long way off this in practice. Wide, rapid variations in airways obstruction are the essence of the definition of asthma. So a proportion of subjects fulfilling the definition of asthma will have normal lung function during a survey. Fortunately for those with airway obstruction it can be measured by simple tests of lung function such as peak expiratory flow rate (PEFR) or forced expiratory volume in one second (FEV_1). These tests are simple and amongst the most reproducible of any lung function tests[6]. Changes in these parameters – either with time (variability) or bronchodilator drugs (reversibility) – are useful in assessing asthma. Although errors are larger than in measuring absolute values, variability and reversibility are still acceptably reproducible.

Bronchial hyper-reactivity can be measured non-invasively by exercise challenge. A fall of more than 15% in PEFR or FEV_1 after a standard exercise test is normally regarded as diagnostic of asthma[5].

Bronchial hyper-reactivity can also be measured by histamine or methacholine challenge. This technique has the advantage of being usable in adults. It is safe and reasonably reproducible and has been used as the basis for several epidemiological surveys[7]. A major problem has been the disparate ways in which results are reported. Some authors report the reduction in PEFR or FEV_1 produced by a specific dose; others the dose of drug required to produce a specific reduction. Thus survey results can be very difficult to compare.

Defining asthma subjectively

In view of the many difficulties outlined above in defining asthma by an objective test, most asthma surveys have been forced to rely on a subjective definition of the disease. The usual criteria are a history of 'wheezing' or the previous diagnosis of 'asthma' by a doctor. However, these two terms mean different things to different people.

The term asthma is often reserved for more severe recurrent episodes of wheezing. These may or may not be associated with respiratory infections. The label 'asthma' is often not applied to these episodes by the subject, unless he/she knows of another person with a similar problem who has been given the label. Doctors have a longstanding disinclination to use the term, especially for children[8]. This underusage appears to be misconstrued and potentially damaging[9]. The term asthma may well be used more frequently for middle-class children[10]. Thus the labelling of asthma by doctors is fairly unreliable and not a good basis for epidemiological survey work when used alone. Wheezing also has a variety of meanings. Almost any type of loud breathing in young children can be described as wheezing. In adults it may also be used to describe the breathing in some varieties of irreversible airways obstruction. Nonetheless the combination of criteria – doctor diagnosis or the presence of wheezing, with some exclusions – probably gives the best working diagnosis available today for survey work.

CLASSIFYING ASTHMA

Asthma is one of the most varied of human diseases. A disease that includes wheezing during a cold in a three-year-old, wheezing only after exercise in a teenager and persistent nocturnal cough in middle age clearly invites attempts to subdivide it. However, classification by these features is unhelpful; we have no evidence that these features imply any differences in the fundamental disease process. Indeed all three disease scenarios above could well occur in the same person as he/she passes through life.

In particular, any attempt to subdivide asthma by time of onset (juvenile or late onset) is simplistic and invalid. Juvenile onset is moderately associated with extrinsic asthma (see later) and late onset with intrinsic asthma. But survey evidence shows that plenty of asthmatics break this rule; juvenile intrinsic asthmatics and late onset extrinsic asthmatics are not uncommon. A similar though less marked disassociation between aetiology and age of onset is currently taking place in diabetes.

Juvenile onset does not equate with extrinsic asthma and late onset does not necessarily imply intrinsic asthma

By far the most logical classification would be by aetiology. But our knowledge of the actual origin of most asthma attacks is so poor that aetiological classification is almost impossible. We can sometimes identify a single cause such as grass pollen exposure in a subject with hay fever or di-isocyanate exposure in a subject with provocation-proven di-isocyanate-induced asthma. But these clear aetiologies comprise only a miniscule proportion of attacks.

We know the cause of asthma attacks only very rarely

There are many hidden assumptions behind how we often view asthma aetiology. These assumptions need further dissection. For instance, there is no evidence that the factors that produce attacks are the same factors which sustain the predisposition to future attacks, manifested by increased bronchial hyper-reactivity. However the commonest assumptions lie behind the most frequent classification – extrinsic or intrinsic asthma.

Extrinsic and intrinsic asthma

These terms were introduced by Rackemann in 1947. He defined extrinsic asthma as being due to 'a clinical sensitiveness to some foreign substance', including food or drug idiosyncracy. Intrinsic asthma was considered non-allergic in origin, caused by infection or 'depletion' after physical or psychic trauma. Today we do not use the terms in quite the same way. Extrinsic asthma now implies asthma with atopy, i.e. with positive skin tests to one or more allergens. Originally, asthma caused by certain compounds such as aspirin, isocyanates and complex platinum salts must have fitted the extrinsic definition. Reactions to these substances are now recognized as non-atopic so are labelled intrinsic. Just as importantly, Rackemann would have required evidence of an actual reaction to an external agent before labelling the asthma extrinsic. Nowadays we only require a positive skin test, even if the patient has no clinical reaction to the agent. This is a sizeable modification. About one-fifth of British schoolchildren have positive skin tests with no evidence of asthma[11]. So about one-fifth of childhood asthmatics could have positive skin tests purely by chance. Are we right to label them as extrinsic? Extrinsic and intrinsic asthma are clinically rather diffuse concepts. We all know examples of the archetypes: the intrinsic asthmatic with onset in middle age, no seasonal variation, relentless deterioration, no response to cromoglycate, etc. and the extrinsic asthmatic with childhood onset, seasonal variation, marked variation over the years, response to cromoglycate and other atopic features such as rhinitis, eczema or drug allergies. But most asthmatics are not at those poles. It seems reasonable to regard asthma as a spectrum with most asthmatics being neither totally extrinsic nor intrinsic[13]. Several genetic studies support this idea. For instance, relatives of intrinsic asthmatics are more likely to have extrinsic than intrinsic asthma[12]. Rather than viewing intrinsic and extrinsic asthma as two unconnected diseases inherited separately, genetic studies suggest that atopy is simply one of various factors increasing the chance that a separately-inherited asthma will be expressed[12,13]. Nonetheless, skin tests are the only objective method we have of classifying asthma. So it seems reasonable to use this method, whatever reservations we have about the real significance of skin tests.

THE PREVALENCE OF ASTHMA

Methods

Asthma surveys are beset by the use of different ways of measuring its frequency of occurrence. The idea of *incidence* is mainly useful for episodic diseases such as measles, rather than recurrent fluctuating diseases like asthma. For asthma one should measure *prevalence*, as:

> *Current prevalence* – the proportion of the survey population who have asthma at the time of the survey.
> *Period prevalence* – the proportion of the population surveyed who have had asthma within a stated period prior to the survey.
> *Cumulative prevalence* – the proportion who have had asthma at any time in their lives.

Cumulative prevalence rates rely heavily on memory, especially for wheezing during childhood. So they are less accurate and are nearly always underestimates. Current prevalence is theoretically more accurate and may be the only parameter suitable for assessing, for instance, variation with time of year or with age. Period prevalence over a short period behaves similarly to current prevalence. Each prevalence gives different results which are difficult to compare. The group surveyed needs to be typical of its population and large enough to reduce sampling errors. However, the more people surveyed, the less information is it feasible to glean from each individual.

An enormous number of surveys of asthma prevalence have been published round the world. The methods used vary greatly in quality – some papers are outstandingly bad. Authors sometimes do not state whether prevalence is current or cumulative, criteria for diagnosing asthma are not given, and so on. One important problem is that many surveys measure the prevalence of atopy, with asthma included only in passing. This type of survey incorrectly presupposes that asthma is only atopic in origin. Credence will only be given below to studies with reasonable, well-defined methodology and no aetiological preconceptions.

Britain

Amongst children, cumulative prevalence has often been surveyed. Rates change from 2.7% in Birmingham schoolchildren[14], 3.5% in a national study[15], 4.8% in Aberdeen schoolchildren[16] to 6.8% in schoolchildren in rural England and Scotland[17]. The weighted average of the best studies is around 3.7%. The results do not vary substantially with exact age range studied or with town/country environment. Current prevalence in children appears remarkably constant with five studies[14,15,18,19] varying only between 1.8% and 2.4%. Only one study[16] gives a higher figure (3.6%).

> Cumulative prevalence in British schoolchildren is about 3.7% with current prevalence around 2%

For adult asthma, a range of good British surveys is available. Cumulative prevalence rates among students range from 3.1% and 3.3% at the University of Wales[20,21] to 5.6% at the University of Cambridge[20]. In the general adult population rates have varied similarly from 3.4% in South Wales[22] to 5.6% in London[23]. As expected a higher cumulative rate of 6.5% has been reported in the elderly[24]. Current prevalence rates are usually between 1.7% and 2.4%[20–22]. The major exception is a large general practice survey in London giving 5.4%[25]. Interestingly, the elderly (70+) gave a fairly high rate of 2.9%[24].

> Child and adult asthma prevalence rates are similar in Britain

The similarity between child and adult current prevalence rates is worth noting. The common image of the asthmatic child growing into the asthma-free adult obviously dominates our thinking too much. In fact adults have as much asthma as children. The approximation between child and adult cumulative prevalence is intriguing, but perhaps partially explicable by the balancing of the competing factors; the adult has longer in which to develop asthmatic attacks and longer to forget them.

> British adults have roughly as much asthma as children

The above rates relate to *asthma*, where the diagnosis was previously made by a doctor or during the survey using specific criteria. If only a history of wheezing episodes is required for inclusion, the rate for *wheeze* will naturally be higher. In British children the cumulative prevalence rate for wheezing appears to be within 11% and 14%, with different studies giving 11%[4], 11.1%[26], and 14.3%[27]. An interesting exception is a follow-up study from birth to 5 years in London, where questioning at regular intervals produced the much higher figure of 24.7%[28]. Thus even cumulative rates among children may be substantial underestimates. Current prevalence of wheezing amongst children has not often been estimated, with one study giving 7.5% among 5–6 year olds[14] and two others 4.3% and 4.9% amongst teenagers[14,15]. Among adults, cumulative prevalence of wheezing has rarely been assessed, with the few results ranging from 12.2%[22] to 24.7%[23].

Thus the British experience is that about 2% of both children and adults currently have asthma and about 3.7% have had asthma at some time. A substantially higher proportion report episodes of wheezing.

Other European Countries

Scandinavia is the only European area for which there is more than scanty data. Cumulative prevalence rates in children used to be low, from 0.7% to 1.8% but all these studies are over 30 years old. In adults, cumulative rates used to range from 1.4% to 2.6% but two more recent surveys have given 3.8% and 4.2%. Thus Scandinavian levels may have been somewhat lower than in Britain in the past, but they seem to have been increasing towards British levels recently. Two French studies have shown similar prevalence levels to Britain. One Dutch study[29] showed much higher levels of both current asthma prevalence and wheezing.

United States

Prevalence rates have been increasing. A large 1928–31 study assessed the asthma prevalence rate in children to be 0.5% for age 5–9 and 0.3% for age 10–14. More recent cumulative rates in children have been 3–4%, roughly the same as in Britain. An interesting study[116] in Houston showed approximately equal rates in white and black children but a much lower rate in Mexican children. The 1928–31 survey[30] in adult showed prevalence rates between 0.1% and 1% depending on age. Again, rates have increased sizeably since then. Recent studies in university students have shown cumulative rates between 3.6% and 5.7%. Probably the largest asthma survey ever was the study by the Public Health Service in 1970[31]. It showed a 12-month prevalence of 3.0%. The survey was based on simply asking subjects if they had asthma. Studies comparing interview surveys and medical records in asthma have shown considerable under-reporting in interviews. If these results are applied to the PHS study then the corrected overall 12-month prevalence is increased to about 4.3%[32]. The PHS survey[31] showed sizeable regional differences within the USA, with increased prevalences in the southern and western regions.

Australasia

Many surveys have been undertaken of cumulative asthma prevalence rates in children in Australia and New Zealand. The rates discovered have ranged from 6% to 19% with most results clustered around 7%. This is of course very much higher than the British average of around 3.7%. One useful study[17] directly compared the cumulative prevalence rates for wheezing in rural schoolchildren in three nations – Britain, Australia and New Zealand. The Australasian rate (10.2%) was substantially higher than the British (6.8%). Asthma surveys among adults have been uncommon although one survey found the high cumulative rate of 12.5% in New Zealand students[33].

Asthma prevalence rates in Australasia are high

Other areas

Africa

The few reliable surveys have shown varying results, but the overall picture is of a very low prevalence of asthma in rural areas and a considerably higher level in town dwellers[34,35].

Asia

India probably has a low prevalence in children, rising slowly with age[36]. Japan appears to have a lowish prevalence of asthma in children although it seems to have risen recently[37].

South America

Virtually no reliable surveys.

Oddities

Tristan da Cunha has a massive cumulative prevalence of 31% in its highly inbred population[38]. The Western Caroline Islands (North of New Guinea) have a similar very high cumulative asthma prevalence of 33%, presumably also due to inbreeding among the population of 240[39]. In contrast, asthma is exceptionally rare among Eskimos[40] and North American Indians[41].

Migration

The study of migrants moving from a low-prevalence area to a high-prevalence area or vice versa should give us useful insights into the relative importance of genetic and environmental factors in the aetiology of asthma. Unfortunately, relatively few studies have been undertaken.

Probably the most helpful studies available are by Morrison Smith *et al.* of English and immigrant schoolchildren in Birmingham[18]. They found relatively low prevalence rates in children born in India and the West Indies, although these were higher than rates in India and the West Indies. However, if the Indian or West Indian children were born in Britain their prevalence rates were similar to those of British children so the longer the exposure to the British environment, the nearer the rate approached the British rate. The study is thus internally consistent in showing a much greater effect of environment than racial predisposition in determining asthma prevalence. A small study in Coventry showed higher prevalence rates for Asian and West Indian children born in Britain than for British children[42]. A survey of matched adult asthma clinic attenders in London[117] showed that Asian immigrants had a later age of onset of asthma – roughly six years later – than British controls. Two-thirds of Asian asthmatics developed asthma after arrival in Britain. Skin test responses were very similar in British and Asian asthmatics. Other migration surveys have tended to bc of highly-inbred isolated communities moving into more urban environments with variable results. Thus most, but not all, migration surveys suggest that asthma prevalence is related more to environment than race.

Studies comprising different ethnic groups living in one area are much harder to interpret, since asthma prevalence may arguably depend on social factors, e.g. income as well as race. For instance, the large American PHS study[31] showed that blacks had a consistently slightly higher asthma prevalence rate than whites. But prevalence was also associated with low income. However, a survey of inner city children in Baltimore[43] showed a higher prevalence in blacks than whites even when the data had been corrected for socio-economic status.

> Studies of migrants and ethnic groups show some possible mild interracial differences but environment is much more important than race in determining asthma prevalence

Using asthma prevalence results

Measuring the prevalence of asthma in a community does not of itself tell us much of immediate practical importance. It can, however, sometimes show communities with very high rates such as in Tristan da Cunha or very low rates such as in rural children. These communities could then be studied further to discover the factors responsible. The main epidemiological interest must be in comparing rates to examine the role of *factors affecting asthma, the natural history of asthma* and *changes in asthma incidence* with time. These will give us valuable insights into the disease, but we should not delude ourselves that we are likely to discover the origin of the disease itself in this way.

FACTORS AFFECTING ASTHMA

Genetic factors

Two types of genetic study have been used: surveying twins and relatives. The definitive twin study is by Edfors-Lubs, who studied 7000 twins in the Swedish Twin Register[44]. She showed that concordance rates were substantially higher in identical twins (19%) than in non-identical twins (4.8%). The concordance rate is the proportion of twin pairs affected by asthma in which both twins have asthma. Thus there is undoubtedly some genetic element in asthma. However, she stresses that both the concordance rates are low and concludes that environment rather than genetics is the dominant factor. A small recent study of 107 twins in Nebraska also showed an increased concordance rate in identical twins[45]. Interestingly, it also confirmed the modest genetic component to methacholine challenge sensitivity and to total IgE levels suggested by previous studies[46,47].

Twin studies show a definite minor genetic element in asthma

Studying relatives of asthmatics can also assess the genetic element in asthma. Asthma has been shown to be commoner in relatives of asthmatics, both in asthma clinic attenders[13] and in general practice[12]. The prevalence of asthma was higher in relatives of extrinsic asthmatics (13%) than in relatives of intrinsic asthmatics (4.5%). If one or both parents also had asthma, the chance of asthma in a sibling is also increased. Similar findings were also noted in an earlier study[48]. Among the relatives of asthmatics, extrinsic asthma was commoner than intrinsic asthma. This was true even for intrinsic asthmatics. At first sight this seems anomalous; why is an intrinsic asthmatic likely to have more extrinsic asthmatics than intrinsic asthmatics in his family? In fact, virtually all the familial results can be encompassed in one hypothesis. Most studies conclude that atopy and asthma are inherited separately. It appears that although atopy does not predispose to asthma, it enhances a genetic susceptibility to asthma. Thus atopy appears to increase the chance that the asthma will be expressed[12,13,48].

> Atopy and asthma are inherited separately. But atopy enhances a genetic susceptibility to asthma, increasing the chance it will be expressed

This group of studies also showed that the family histories of asthma were remarkably similar for children who had asthma or wheezy bronchitis[49]. This suggests that asthma and wheezy bronchitis are probably essentially the same disease. Three clinical studies[3,4,9] also suggest that this is correct. The inheritance of asthma is likely to be either dominant with incomplete penetrance or more likely polygenic[12,13,44].

Atopy

Until fairly recently asthma was almost always seen as purely an allergic phenomenon. Indeed, in many recent surveys it is still being thought of in this way. However, with more detailed investigation the phenomenon of intrinsic or skin-test-negative asthma has emerged. The role of atopy in asthma pathogenesis has been increasingly questioned. The genetic studies outlined above have contributed the important realisation that asthma and atopy are inherited separately. Nonetheless, subjects born with an asthmatic predisposition are more likely to have that predisposition expressed if they are also atopic.

If atopy acts as a 'forcing factor' in the expression of asthma, one would expect extrinsic asthma to be expressed earlier than intrinsic disease. This appears to be the case. Asthmatics with onset at age below 10 usually have greater skin test responses[50]. Another study found that 50% of extrinsic asthmatics had onset before age 18, whereas only 13% of intrinsic asthmatics had done so[51].

In an Australian study[52] of 11,551 asthmatics, the disease appeared to be intrinsic in a substantial majority of the youngest (less than 4 years old) and oldest (age over 60) cases. Asthma was more likely to be extrinsic at other ages, especially the 15–29 year-old group where the proportion reached 83%. However, all studies agree that there are many exceptions to the early-onset-extrinsic, late-onset-intrinsic trend. A 73-year-old new-onset extrinsic asthmatic and a 7-year-old intrinsic asthmatic are mildy uncommon but they are not rarities.

Extrinsic asthma tends to start early in life but there are exceptions

Atopy seems to be moderately associated with wheezy bronchitis, but less than with childhood asthma. A study in London[53] found that children with wheezy bronchitis were more likely to have positive skin tests than controls but less likely to have positive skin tests than asthmatics. A study in Melbourne[3] found a similar incidence of positive skin tests in wheezy bronchitis and asthma but did not test for house-dust mite – a very common childhood allergen. Asthma is associated with other atopic diseases. In a survey in Michigan allergic rhinitis was about six times commoner in asthmatics than in the general population[54]. A national survey in Britain found that hay-fever was seven times commoner if children also had asthma[15]. In Iowa, 78% of extrinsic asthmatics also had allergic rhinitis and 38% of patients with allergic rhinitis also had wheezing[55,56].

Eczema is also strongly associated with asthma. In Melbourne, 14% of mildly asthmatic children had eczema, rising to 83% of severe cases[57]. Severity of the two diseases was associated. Conversely, between 20% and 60% of patients with eczema also have asthma[58].

Both allergic rhinitis and eczema are also commoner in the families of asthmatics[13]. This is obvious for extrinsic asthmatics, but the data also suggests a slight tendency for this also to be true for intrinsic asthmatics. This slightly odd finding is in keeping with the theory outlined above for the genetic links between asthma and atopy. Bendixen has pointed out that rhinitis and asthma have many clinical features in common, regardless of the role of atopy[59]. Atopic subjects are more likely to develop allergic symptoms when they encounter an allergen they have not previously met. In an interesting study Frankland showed that 25% of those with a history of hay fever developed rhinitis or asthma on starting to work with locusts in a laboratory[60]. The comparable figure for non-atopics was only 5%. Thus atopy may well be a risk factor for developing occupational asthma.

Atopy may well be a risk factor for occupational asthma

Extrinsic asthma is associated with the production of high levels of specific IgE. This has been well documented in several studies[61,62]. High levels of non-specific IgE have been shown in rural Third World populations with high intestinal parasite loads[35,63]. It has been postulated that the high levels of non-specific IgE might competitively displace specific IgE from mast cell IgE receptor sites. This could explain the low levels of asthma found in these areas[35]. However, a survey in Nigeria[64] gives results which are incompatible with this concept. Parasite infestations were just as frequent in asthmatics as in controls. No association was found between skin test results and total IgE levels and IgE levels were similar in urban and rural environments. Thus the low asthma prevalence and high non-specific IgE levels found in rural Africa may be more coincidental than causal.

The presence of atopy does not increase bronchial reactivity unless asthma itself is present[65]. This is of course compatible with the theory outlined previously that asthma and atopy are inherited separately. The role of atopy in asthma deaths has been studied[66] and will be described in more detail later. Atopy was particularly associated with sudden onset and rapid death. Atopic deaths tended to be in younger patients and to occur during peak months for extrinsic asthmatic attacks.

Climate

Much has been written on climate and asthma, often with contradictory conclusions. Various factors – overall climate, season, altitude, pollen and spore counts and personal micro-environment – are so intertwined that valid firm conclusions are often impossible. Nonetheless, there is reasonable evidence suggesting that asthma is commoner in damp than dry climates. Asthma is also probably rarer above 2000–2500 metres altitude.

Cullen has studied rural schoolchildren in Britain, Australia and New Zealand[17]. The children were almost all of similar ethnic origin. Contrary to popular prejudice, the warmer the region the higher was the prevalence of asthma. Overall cumulative asthma prevalence was 10% in Australia and New Zealand and 7% in Britain. Another minor surprise was that asthma prevalence was actually lower in areas with high summer rainfall. The same results were found for childhood bronchitis and hay fever. No association was found with winter rainfall.

The important role that micro-environment can play has been shown in Hong Kong[67]. Peak months for asthma and allergic rhinitis are November to January. The months coincide with a peak in monthly specific IgE for house-dust mite. At this time there is increased use of bedding quilts which are not used during the summer. A parallel role for house-dust mite in blankets has been suggested to explain the rapid rise in asthma in the Papua New Guinea highlands[68]. So your own micro-climate can occasionally make a considerable difference.

Asthma is commoner in hotter, damper climates

Season

In 400 BC Hippocrates noted that asthma was more common and apt to be worse in the autumn[69]. Since then this seasonal variation has been well documented round the world. Hospital admissions for childhood asthma in England and Wales show a consistent monthly pattern[70]. There are two annual peaks – in early summer (June–July) and early autumn (September). The same pattern is shown in the Royal College of General Practitioners' survey of the weekly incidence of asthmatic attacks[71]. This bimodal pattern appears all round the world. In Britain the early summer peak is well correlated with grass pollen counts[71] in each year. The autumn peak correlates with a rise in acute bronchitis notifications in children[70] and may well be related to the seasonal rise in respiratory viral infections[72,73]. The house-dust mite population also rises in autumn and this could also be related[74]. Spectacular autumn 'epidemics' of asthma sometimes occur in the United States, especially in New Orleans and New York[75]. They do not appear to be related to peaks of atmospheric pollution. It is curious that reports consistently show a sizeable midwinter trough and a smaller midsummer trough. Their cause is unknown.

Asthmatic attacks are most common in early summer and in autumn

Month of birth

Several studies have tried to link asthma with month of birth but their results are so diverse that there appears to be no genuine association.

Infection

The role of 'infection' in precipitating acute exacerbations in chronic asthma is well known and documented. But infections may also cause the onset of asthma or wheezy bronchitis. A longitudinal study of children[73] has shown that 8% of normal children developed wheezing for the first time with a para-influenza virus infection and 25% with a rhinovirus infection. Most of these children had further attacks of wheezy bronchitis and some went on to overt asthma. In a study of adults with late-onset asthma, 47% described their first episode of wheezing as being due to a respiratory infection[76].

Infection can precipitate the first attack of asthma

Psyche

For a long time asthma has been vaguely associated with an anxious, neurotic personality with suppressed resentment. However this popular prejudice is not valid. Many surveys have assessed personality traits in asthmatics according to a large range of parameters[77–79]. The evidence is quite unequivocal; there is no association between asthma and any known personality trait.

There is no specific asthmatic personality

Asthma is not a psychomatic disease. An asthmatic's level of wheezing can be moderately affected by emotional upset but this is also true of many other diseases such as angina never considered to be psychomatic.

THE NATURAL HISTORY OF ASTHMA

The overall natural history of asthma is poorly defined. It is difficult to assess because it requires prospective studies of large numbers of subjects for long periods. The diagnostic criteria used are particularly critical and frequently cause problems.

One of the earliest large-scale studies was by Rackemann and Edwards[80], who followed 440 subjects with onset of asthma before age 13 for an average of 20 years. Half the patients became totally symptom-free during follow-up and another quarter had no wheezing if they avoided their allergens. Negative skin tests were strongly associated with complete remission. Almost every study of childhood asthma shows a preponderance of boys. Rackemann and Edwards[80] found that sex did not alter prognosis but most studies have found that boys are more likely to have remissions than girls so the preponderance of boys declines through adolescence. However, boys remain predominant in the more severe grades[81]. More severe asthma in earlier childhood is less likely to remit completely during adolescence but the symptoms improve in about half the more severe patients between 14 and 21 years of age[81].

At least 75% of childhood asthmatics have little or no asthma by age 21

Despite this substantial overall improvement in asthma with increasing age, Martin *et al.* found that recurrences were not uncommon during adolescence[81]. At age 21 spirometric lung function was normal in all but the most severe grades but most subjects still had bronchial hyper-reactivity. Even amongst those who had not wheezed for over three years some 60% still had bronchial hyper-reactivity at the age of 21[82].

The Tecumseh study[54] showed that remissions were also common in adult asthma, with the peak four year remission rates for any age group occurring in young adult males (age 16–44) and older women (age over 45). However, the short four year interval is inadequate to show them to be permanent remissions.

Remissions are common in adult asthma

The effect of other atopic features on prognosis has been studied. Allergic rhinitis and positive skin tests probably have little effect, but childhood eczema is probably associated with more persistent asthma. The great majority of patients who have both hay fever and asthma developed asthma first, or developed both diseases within a few months of each other. Thus using hyposensitization for hay fever in the hope of preventing asthma is very unlikely to be effective[54].

Eczema in childhood is associated with more persistent asthma but allergic rhinitis and positive allergen skin tests are not

Only 5–10% of hay fever sufferers develop asthma

TRENDS IN THE PREVALENCE OF ASTHMA

Anecdotal evidence strongly suggests that asthma has become commoner in the last few decades. But has it? If it has, is this just caused by greater awareness or diagnostic fashion? Is the asthma becoming more severe as well? Epidemiological studies have addressed these questions from several different angles.

Hospital admission rates for asthma in England and Wales doubled between 1959 and 1963[83]. An 'epidemic' of asthma deaths occurring at the same time as rising bronchodilator aerosol sales was first noticed in 1965. It will be discussed below, but the previous rise in hospital admissions cannot be attributed to heightened anxiety among general practitioners or hospital staff. The same substantial rise was found in children; Anderson noted a threefold increase in childhood asthma admission rates between 1959 and 1973[84]. Springett found that during this period there was no increase in days off work certified as being due to asthma[83]. Thus the incidence of asthma attacks appeared to remain static but more of the attacks were severe enough to require admission.

After the peak of the asthma 'epidemic' in the mid-sixties, hospital admission rates and asthma deaths declined to the levels of the late-fifties. This removed much of the incentive for the search to find a convincing explanation for the mid-sixties peak. During the early seventies admission and death rates remained at roughly the late-fifties levels. This was regarded with satisfaction and possibly complacency. However in the last decade, since the mid-seventies, a worrying increasing trend in admissions and deaths is beginning to be seen again. Monthly admissions for childhood asthma tripled in the period 1975–81[70]. By far the greatest percentage rise in admissions came in the very young below 5 years old. There was a steady upward trend in adult asthma admissions during 1974–84[85]. These rises are unlikely to be caused by changes in diagnostic fashion[70,86].

Asthma deaths will be discussed in detail later but their time trends are relevant here. After the 1964–66 'epidemic', deaths fell sharply in 1967–69 and by 1970 had returned to the 1960 level. There was a further gratifying reduction through 1971–75 reaching a nadir in 1975[87]. Since then there has been a gradual increase averaging 4.7% per annum[88]. This increase is virtually all in the 5–34 year age group, with the 35–64 year age group virtually unchanged. The rise in male deaths is slightly faster – 6.1% per annum. These increases are unlikely to be statistical artefacts[88].

> After the asthma peak of the mid-1960s hospital admissions and deaths declined until 1975. Since then the rates have been climbing steadily

A steep rise in asthma mortality since 1974 has recently been reported from New Zealand. There the post-epidemic drop in mortality had been slow, with the 1974 rate still twice the pre-epidemic level. Since 1974 the death rate in the 5–34 age group has *tripled* to well above the epidemic peak and six times the rate for England and Wales. This massive rise fortunately appears to be limited to New Zealand and is being investigated vigorously in a national study of all asthma deaths[90]. Asthma deaths in the United States have also started to increase, rising 75% between 1975 and 1983[91].

New Zealand has recently had a huge rise in asthma deaths

Hospital admissions and death rates only provide indirect information about the incidence of the most severe forms of asthma. To find if their recent rising trend is typical of all grades of asthma we need community based surveys. The best type of survey would require sequential study of current prevalence using an identical survey technique on each occasion. Such a survey is not available. Morrison Smith *et al.* noted a 30% increase in the current prevalence of asthma in Birmingham schoolchildren between 1957 and 1975[14,18], although the survey methods varied slightly between the two studies. More recent data have come from the Royal College of General Practitioners Research Unit. Each week this unit monitors the number of patients consulting their general practitioners for specific diseases. Participating practices are broadly distributed throughout England and Wales. The one-week prevalence of asthma increased substantially from 10.2 per 1000 population in 1970 to 18.2 per 1000 in 1981[92]. This shows an 80% rise in 11 years. The increase appears to be real and not to be caused by diagnostic preference. A further publication shows that the high 1981 rates have persisted up to 1983[71]. Because of the size of the survey this is powerful evidence of a substantial recent increase in asthma prevalence in the community.

Asthma consultations in general practice rose by 80% between 1970 and 1981

Thus all parameters – asthma deaths, hospital admissions and community prevalence – have been rising in recent years.

However there is a gradation; mild asthma (GP consultations) shows a large rise, more severe asthma (hospital admissions) a moderate rise and the most severe asthma (deaths) a smaller rise. The bulk of the increase in asthma therefore appears to have been at the milder end of the spectrum.

ASTHMA DEATHS

Background

Each year about 2300 people die from asthma in England and Wales[88]. About 600 of these are in the 5–34 age group. As noted above the death rate fell slightly during the early 1970s but since 1975 it has been rising again. Asthma deaths in the 5–34 age group doubled between 1977 and 1983[87]. Every one of these deaths is a tragedy which in theory should be preventable. We need to examine asthma deaths closely to find out how these tragedies can be avoided in the future.

> Asthma kills about 2300 people every year in England and Wales. Some 600 deaths are below the age of 35

First we need to know if we can rely on asthma death statistics. They depend on the accuracy of death certificates. The most detailed study of accuracy was done by the British Thoracic Society[93] who examined death certificates mentioning 'asthma' in two regions of England in 1979. They concluded that death certificates overestimated asthma deaths by 13%. Ormerod and Stableforth found an overestimate of 15% in Birmingham[94]. Accuracy is highest in the younger age groups. Thus death certificates for asthma are in fact more accurate than for many other acute diseases[93]. A similar high level of accuracy has been found in New Zealand[89].

> Asthma death figures are reliable because death certificates for asthma are normally accurate

Age

Death rates rise strongly with age in a smooth and almost exponential fashion. The rate from the age of one to 45 rises slowly, only roughly tripling in this period. Then it gradually speeds up, with the rate for age 85+ some twelve times that at age 45[91]. Even if death certification in the elderly is less accurate this is still a formidable rise. Although attention is understandably focused on younger asthma deaths it should not be forgotten that 75% of people dying from asthma are over the age of 35. The average age of death in our Cardiff asthma death surveys[95,96] was 49 years.

Most asthma deaths occur in the middle-aged and elderly

Sex

Sex does not influence death rates substantially. In England and Wales death rates for males and females are roughly equal, with a variable minimal preponderance of males in recent years. In the USA every year from 1968 to 1980 has shown a slight excess of females[91]. Within these overall figures there is a tendency for male deaths to be slightly younger.

Atopy

Atopy influences asthma deaths. Our Cardiff study[95,96] found that 48% of the deaths were atopic and the BTA study of 90 deaths[66] found a figure of 60%. They found that the final attack tended to be more rapidly progressive in atopics. They were also more likely to die in the seasonal May/June and September/October peaks. Atopics tended to die younger (average age 40 compared to 52 for non-atopics) but had had asthma for much longer. A curious finding was that half the atopic patients died at weekends whereas for non-atopic patients deaths were distributed evenly throughout the week.

Despite the association between juvenile asthma and atopy over 40% of deaths in the 5–19 age group were not atopic. So young severe asthmatics are not always atopic.

> Half of asthma deaths are in atopics. They tend to die younger and have more rapid fatal attacks

Time of death

Much emphasis was given to diurnal variation in the airways obstruction in asthma a few years ago. One would thus expect most asthmatics to die at night. A modest excess of nocturnal deaths has been found in the BTA[97] and the New Zealand nebuliser[98] studies as well as some smaller studies. However, both the Birmingham[94] and Cardiff[95,96] studies showed no significant trend towards deaths at night. So it appears that if there is a tendency to die at night it is not large.

Season

Asthmatics are more likely to die in late summer with August deaths 45% above the monthly average. This contrasts strongly with the marked drop in hospital admissions for asthma seen in August[70]. Summer holidays must disrupt normal patterns of asthma care. One might speculate that in holiday periods more severe asthma might be tolerated for longer. This would bring a drop in admissions and an increase in deaths, especially if unfamiliarity delayed medical referral. There is no death peak coinciding with the early summer grass pollen season. Deaths are at their lowest in midwinter unlike most other diseases.

> More asthmatics than expected die in late summer and fewer in midwinter

Before the fatal attack

Before examining the fatal attack itself we need to try to see what led up to it. We need to examine the patient's overall disease – its history as well as its management by both doctor and patient.

Asthma history

The age of onset of asthma was examined in the BTA study[66]. Just over half had onset before age 15 but 25% had onset after the age of 35. In the Cardiff study[96] only 30% of hospital deaths had started asthma before the age of 20 and 48% started after age 40. These slightly differing figures both suggest that asthma that kills tends to start in childhood or in middle age. The duration of asthma history varies widely from one month to 63 years[94,96]. However, virtually all were chronic asthmatics with only 2%[95] or 9%[66] dying within 5 years of onset. The majority had had asthma for over 20 years[66]. The mean duration is agreed to be long: 16.5 years[94], 17.5 years[95,96] and about 22 years[66] in different series.

Asthma deaths tend to be in long-standing chronic asthmatics

Previous asthma admissions[66,94–96,110]

Two-thirds of deaths had previously had sufficiently severe asthma to require hospital admission. The figure of 66–68% is remarkably constant in all series. Between 15% and 27% had had multiple admissions. In the year before death between 22% and 38% had been admitted. Perhaps the most poignant statistic is that roughly 12% had actually been discharged from hospital less than one month before dying of asthma. In some series a smaller proportion had even been discharged less than one week before death. Thus recent hospital discharge by no means guarantees good asthma control.

> Two-thirds of asthma deaths had been in hospital before for their asthma – roughly one-third in their last year of life

In contrast the BTA study[66] showed that one-third of patients had had no asthma at all for at least three months of their last year. In New Zealand the figure is much lower (9%)[110].

Recent severity of asthma

The BTA study[66] found that throughout the last month of life 62% of patients had been able to work, 33% with no difficulty. Only 10% had been on chronic sick leave because of asthma. Thus although the group usually had long-standing asthma, they were surprisingly healthy. So good adaptation and no recent invalidity does not preclude imminent death.

Previous management by general practitioner

For good management of asthma, the general practitioner must actually diagnose asthma, appreciate the disease severity, prescribe adequate therapy, monitor its efficacy and in most cases have the disease assessed by a specialist outpatient clinic. Similar criteria apply to hospital outpatient supervision. The most detailed assessment of GP care in the last month of life is the BTA study[66,100]. Its results are a damning indictment. Some aspects of management or supervision were deficient in virtually all cases (88 out of 90). In a small number of cases asthma was never actually diagnosed. More frequent follow-up was indicated in 78% of deaths, the patient's deterioration was not appreciated in 63%, serial lung function tests such as peak flow were required but not undertaken in 92% and so on. From detailed interviews with the dead patient's GP and relatives, there was little evidence that patients or relatives were adequately instructed in the use of steroids, especially for exacerbations of asthma, or what to do in severe attacks. Although the retrospectoscope is a powerful instrument, the standards used in this study were reasonable and easily attainable. British general practice comes out badly from this study.

Chronic asthmatics need *much* more GP supervision, especially with unstable asthma. Peak flows are mandatory

The survey also shows for the first time a problem caused by change of general practitioner. Patients were considered to have changed their GPs too often in 21% of deaths. Seven percent had changed GPs within six weeks of death. Very similar figures were found in New Zealand[110]. So continuity of care seems to be important. How many other patients have poor continuity from seeing different partners in a large practice or from seeing a stream of registrars in clinics?

Continuity of care is important for severe asthmatics

With the dominant pattern of substantial long-standing asthma noted previously it is surprising that between one-third and one-half of the patients who later died had never been referred to an outpatient clinic[94–96].

Previous management by hospital clinic

Only one quarter of patients were under regular hospital supervision[66]. The BTA study is also scathing about the quality of outpatient care. Serial lung function tests were needed but not performed in 88% of deaths, more frequent follow-up was indicated in 65% and the patient's deterioration was not noticed in 30%. Overall hospital outpatient care was deficient in virtually all cases (96%). The Cardiff study of deaths outside hospital[95] paints a similar gloomy picture with only half the patients having necessary lung function tests at clinics.

Routine drug treatment[66,94–96,110]

The vast majority of patients were taking bronchodilators. Many used inhalers but in two studies about half the patients used oral bronchodilators, which are much less efficient, are markedly slower in action and have many more side-effects. The timing of the surveys suggests that the use of this inefficient form of treatment might be declining. Certainly sales of inhaled bronchodilators are increasing[101].

Theophyllines were taken by 40% of patients in the BTA study. However, only about half the patients were on regular oral steroids before the final attack (49%, 50% and 56% in three studies). This low percentage is made more alarming by the low dosages found in all studies. Only in 10% of all patients studied were they taking more than 10 mg prednisolone per day. Of all drugs, only steroids will reverse the mucosal oedema and bronchial plugging which are dominant features of moderate or severe asthma. All studies have commented on this dangerous underuse of larger prednisolone doses. It must be a major cause of the events leading up to death from asthma. To contribute to an asthma patient's continual misery or even death by using inadequate steroid doses because of half-remembered vague fears of osteoporosis is plain bad medical care. Patients are much more likely to die of asthma than steroids. Most chest clinics see sizeable numbers of asthmatics who have needed 20–25 mg prednisolone daily for years to control their asthma. There is nothing unusual or excessive in these dosages. The right dose of steroid is the minimum to give good control. If that is 30 mg per day then give 30 mg per day.

> Far too few asthma deaths have had oral steroids, and steroid doses were far too timid

Drug treatment in the month before death

In the month prior to the final attack the BTA survey[66] felt that bronchodilator dosage should have been increased in 20% of patients and bronchodilators started in a further 7%. Half the patients taking oral steroids needed a larger dose and an additional 12% should have started them. Overall treatment was satisfactory in 40% but increased treatment was needed in 60%. In the Cardiff study four of 36 patients on prednisolone had their dosage increased in their last month, while

10 actually had their dose reduced[95]. In Birmingham, 37% of patients attended their GP in the last two weeks before their death but in none was their therapy significantly altered. Thus the problems of underuse and underdosage seen with routine drug treatment were accentuated during their last month of life, and GPs often failed to appreciate the deterioration in their patients' asthma.

> In the month before death most patients needed more treatment from their GPs

Patient compliance

The best-planned asthma treatment in the world is no use if the patient does not do what he is told. One study has assessed patient compliance in the year before death[66] and found that only half the patients co-operated well. The commonest failure was reluctance or refusal to summon medical help and one quarter of patients were unreliable in taking their drugs. One patient in eight defaulted from medical care.

It might be comforting to blame the patient alone for these compliance problems, but that is not the whole story. Compliance is a complex field. Research has shown that medical attitudes and perceptiveness strongly influence patient compliance[102]. Since the same study[66] showed poor counselling in the use of steroids and what to do in an emergency, other aspects of counselling were probably poor as well. Asthma is not an easy disease for doctors to explain. Treatment is not very easy to take in at first glance. Explanation takes time and thought. Poor patient compliance is the result of a failure in the doctor–patient relationship. That failure is not often totally the patient's fault, however much we would wish to project our own failings on to him.

> Half the patients who die of asthma do not comply well with medical advice. Poor compliance can often be partly the doctor's fault.

The Fatal Attack

Assessment of the sequence of events before death depends critically on the speed of onset of the final attack.

Speed of onset

Medical perceptions of the speed of onset of a fatal asthma attack have changed recently. An episode of severe asthma used always to be a matter of days or even weeks as implied by the term 'status asthmaticus'. However, in 1968 Speizer *et al.*[103] examined asthma deaths in the 1966–67 'epidemic'. They found that 28% had died within one hour of the start of the attack, 56% within six hours and 70% within 24 hours. A further more detailed survey[104] by the same group in 1968–69, after the 'epidemic' had passed, recorded a slightly lower proportion of short attack durations: 16% after less than one hour and 60% after less than 24 hours. The emphasis at this time was on bronchodilator aerosols and the short duration of most fatal attacks was not emphasized. The clinical importance of rapidly fatal attacks was perhaps first heavily emphasized in the 1977 Cardiff study of deaths outside hospital[95]. Twenty-three percent died in the first 30 minutes. Other studies[66,94,98,110] have noted 19%, 23%, 24% and 26% of deaths occurring in the first hour. All studies agree that a substantial majority of deaths occur in the first 24 hours – 67%[94], 78%[95], and 81%[66]. The BTA study[66] usefully pointed out that patients with a history of severe, rapidly progressing attacks were particularly likely to die rapidly; 43% of them died within one hour and virtually all within 24 hours.

> One quarter of asthma deaths occur within an hour of the start of the attack; three-quarters die within 24 hours.

Deaths in hospital seem to be rather different – the fatal attack is much longer. The Cardiff study of 53 hospital deaths[96] showed that only 19% died within 24 hours and the final episode lasted more than four days in the majority of patients.

Two other smaller studies[66,94] have given a similar picture. The difference is too substantial to be explained simply by the time taken to transfer to hospital. Perhaps hospital treatment at least slows down the decline to death and hopefully enables an unknown number to escape death and recover.

Hospital deaths have often had wheezing for more than four days

Non-fatal episodes of acute severe asthma tend to be between hospital and non-hospital deaths in speed of onset, defined as the period from the start of the attack to the summoning of medical help[105]. This fits in well with the observation for asthma deaths that, where GPs were called in, half the patients were dead or moribund when they arrived[66]. Thus underestimation of the final attack and fatal delay by the patient could well be an important factor. Although the recent emphasis has been on rapid death in asthmatics it is important not to let this pendulum swing too far and fatalism set in. There is a broad spectrum of fatal attack duration. We must remember that half the fatal attacks last at least eight hours[95]; even this is a long time if patients realize not to delay in summoning assistance and prompt effective treatment is given.

Encourage patients to seek help sooner

Unavoidable deaths

There is a 'hard core' of asthmatics who die rapidly despite appropriate treatment before and during the final attack – 25% in a New Zealand study[98] and 11% in the BTA study[66]. A larger group die within 30 minutes or one hour of onset. They probably cannot be saved during the acute attack but some of these attacks might be prevented by better long-term care.

Only about 1 asthma death in 10 is unavoidable

The BTA study[66] found that about 90% of asthma deaths were potentially preventable. Apart from problems with care before the attack, failures during the final attack fall into the three groups discussed below.

Severity of attack not appreciated by the patient

The BTA panel felt that 77% of patients at home delayed sending for medical help probably because they did not appreciate the severity of the asthma attack. Why do they do this? It is well-known that asthma is almost too easy a disease to live with, when the asthmatic has forgotten what it is like not to be breathless. Some asthmatics undoubtedly do have reduced perception of breathlessness. Rubinfield and Pain[106] found that even when severe airways obstruction had been induced by methacholine, 15% of asthmatics had no symptoms of dyspnoea. Perception of breathlessness seems to be less in asthmatics with chronic airways obstruction and in those asthmatics with greater reactivity to histamine[107]. This failure of perception exists among those whose asthma starts only in middle age and those who only have occasional attacks as well as among lifelong asthmatics. A further factor may be that those who have developed and survived severe acute attacks before do not consider the possibility of death and do not summon medical assistance.

Some asthmatics seriously underestimate how ill they are

Severity of attack not appreciated by doctor

The BTA study panel felt that the attending doctor had failed to appreciate the severity of the asthma in 70% of patients at home and 23% of patients in hospital[66]. This assessment dovetails with the Cardiff evidence that of 21 seen still alive only 12 were recommended for hospital admission by their

GPs[95]. The comparable figure for the Birmingham study[94] was only two patients out of 11. No patient had an objective lung function measurement made. Why do doctors not recognize life-threatening asthma? Asthma *in extremis* can look radically different to the distressed tachypnoeic patient with noisy respiration we all recognize as typical of acute severe asthma. The patient near death may be tired, not severely distressed and have a quiet chest. He may look subdued but often has a severe tachycardia. The danger signs are quiet chest and tachycardia. The best objective test is peak flow which is as easily measured as blood pressure.

Your long-standing asthmatic with no rhonchi could well be very very *ill*. Measure his pulse and peak flow.

In the final phase of the fatal attack wheezy respiration was found in less than 10% of patients. It was usually described as gasping, gulping or retching respiration[100].

Hospital doctors can also fail to assess their patients properly. Patients dying in general medical wards have usually had their lung function measured on admission and almost never thereafter[94,96]. Serial peak flow measurements are mandatory for adequate care. Arterial blood gases should be measured on every admission with acute severe asthma. There are two broad categories of hospital death[96]. Firstly, those who are half-dead on arrival and decline inexorably to death. Secondly, those who make a good initial partial recovery but have persistent tachycardia and die later. The 40% of hospital deaths in the latter category virtually die of neglect.

Bad medical management is a major cause of hospital asthma deaths

Inadequate treatment

General practitioners often give patients inadequate treatment in the final attack. In the Cardiff series[95] treatment details are known in 12 patients. Three were given intravenous aminophylline, three subcutaneous adrenaline and three oral steroids. Two had no change made in their previous regimen. Even where oral steroids were used the immediate doses given were prednisolone 5 mg or 10 mg, to be repeated three times daily. No patient received intravenous steroids. Slightly worse treatment was given in the later Birmingham series[94]. The treatment in the slightly more recent BTA study[66] was no better, with inadequate or no treatment being given in 25 out of 30 patients seen alive by general practitioners.

Hospital doctors' initial treatment is better but sometimes barely adequate. In the first two hours after admission only two-thirds of patients had been given any form of steroids[96]. Three-quarters received intravenous aminophylline, but less than one-quarter had an intravenous infusion set up. By 24 hours after admission average treatment had improved but 15% had still received less than 400 mg hydrocortisone, 17% less than 20 mg prednisolone and 4% had received no treatment at all. Similar results were found in Birmingham[94], where it was noted that no patient had ever received nebulized or intravenous bronchodilator. Five of fifteen patients were given sedatives.

Inadequate immediate treatment causes asthma deaths

What treatment should be given to a patient seen in life-threatening asthma? Obviously the first requirement to prevent death is intravenous steroids, usually 200 mg hydrocortisone. A bronchodilator for immediate relief could either be aminophylline or preferably intravenous or nebulized salbutamol/terbutaline. Aminophylline is now being used less in hospital since it adds nothing to frequent nebulized salbutamol/terbutaline. It is still useful in general practice but it is important never to use it in patients taking sustained release theophyllines. The usual starting dose of aminophylline is 250 mg by slow intravenous injection. Nowadays slow intravenous salbutamol (250 mcg) or terbutaline (250 mcg) are considered as effective and less toxic. Probably the best immediate relief is by nebulized salbutamol or terbutaline (2.5–5 mg in 5 ml saline or one proprietary Nebule or Respule). Nebulizers only cost £75 each and every practice should have one.

In life-threatening asthma in general practice use immediately:

200 mg IV hydrocortisone, plus
- 250 mg slow IV aminophylline, or
- 250 mcg slow IV salbutamol, or
- 2.5 mg nebulized salbutamol

Delay in medical assistance

Both GPs and ambulances arrived promptly in the BTA study, with two-thirds of local GPs and three-quarters of ambulances arriving within 15 minutes. Deputising services were much slower; only 38% arrived in the first half-hour. The Cardiff study also found no evidence of delay. So delay in the arrival of medical assistance summoned in life-threatening asthma is not a significant factor in asthma deaths.

Can treatment cause death?

Although inadequate assessment, delay and inadequate treatment are clearly the most important avoidable factors in asthma deaths we also need to consider whether deaths can be caused by the treatment itself. The question was first raised in the 1964–65 asthma 'epidemic' in Britain. Here a sudden steep increase in asthma deaths coincided with the rapidly rising use of isoprenaline inhalers. Initially the reasonable assumption was made that the inhalers were causing the epidemic and over-the-counter inhalcr sales were banned. Inhaler sales fell rapidly as did asthma deaths. Obviously the case was proven. But was it? Gandevia[108] found that a similar rise and fall in asthma deaths occurred in Australia despite rapidly rising inhaler sales throughout. In fact, well over twice as many inhalers were being sold when asthma deaths were falling as when deaths were rising. The Australian experience and other evidence[109] made a direct link between inhalers and deaths unlikely. Over the years since then an international consensus view of the 1960s epidemic has gradually emerged. In the mid-1960s the introduction of sympathomimetic inhalers transformed most asthmatics' lives. So in a severe attack they tried to rely more and more on them, but got less and less relief. The ensuing delay in summoning assistance and the underuse of steroids were probably what caused the wave of deaths. Publicity of the danger of death in asthma attacks, the 'danger' of excessive inhaler use and the realization that inhalers were ineffective in severe attacks all caused asthmatics to call for help earlier. Deaths then declined. No one cause is likely to account fully for the epidemic but the above appears to fit most of the facts.

Isoprenaline inhalers probably did not cause the 1960s deaths epidemic

Selective sympathomimetic bronchodilators such as salbutamol and terbutaline were introduced following the epidemic and there is no evidence to link them with any changes in the asthma death rate. Sales have risen inexorably throughout the 1970s as the asthma rate first fell gradually to 1975 then subsequently rose.

Salbutamol/terbutaline inhalers appear to be safe

But the ghost of the 1960s epidemic still haunts us. Inhalers are still regarded by non-specialists as in some way vaguely dangerous. Manufacturers still print 'it is dangerous to exceed the recommended dose' on inhalers, doubtless at the behest of their overcautious legal departments. GPs still restrict inhaler use too much. After all, one standard nebulizer dose is the equivalent of 25–50 puffs of aerosol, so a nebulizer patient will often be on the equivalent of 200 puffs of aerosol daily. If patients require to use their inhalers very frequently the underlying treatment needs to be increased. A spectacular rise in asthma deaths occurred in New Zealand in 1977–79[89] and the high death rate has persisted. In young adults the rate is some 5–6 times that in Britain. Fortunately this rise has not occurred elsewhere. It has been suggested that the combination of high-dose sympathomimetic bronchodilators and oral theophyllines is contributing to the increase in deaths[111] but this has been disputed[112]. The increasing role of nebulizers has been suggested as a possible reason[113]. However, a new study of nebulizer deaths in New Zealand[98] has found similar circumstances for death to those found in previous non-nebulizer studies. Nebulizers do not in themselves seem to be dangerous, but undue faith in them can bring fatal delay in seeking assistance. Over-reliance on nebulizers was considered to be a major factor in only 8% of asthma deaths. This could not explain the recent tripling of asthma deaths.

Sales of all asthma drugs increased sharply in 1979–80 in New Zealand but this is well after the rise in deaths in 1975–77 and so is likely to be a response to the deaths rather than a cause of them. No convincing explanation has yet been put forward for the wave of deaths confined to New Zealand. It may be partially due to a genuine increase in asthma severity[110]. In the ongoing research epidemiology is a major tool.

> In the present New Zealand asthma deaths epidemic nebulizers may play a minor role but the main reason is still unknown

Prevention of asthma deaths

Prevention of home deaths centres on two aspects: quality of basic care and delay. The quality of previous care found in patients dying of asthma is normally poor, and in some cases downright awful. We have good drugs for asthma – bronchodilator aerosols, aerosol and oral steroids with sometimes theophyllines and cromoglycate. What we need to do is *use them*. In a magnificent thundering editorial in Thorax, Seaton[114] has pointed out that in almost no other field is the gap between diagnostic and therapeutic knowledge and its general application so great. The principles of diagnosis and treatment are so simple. But misconceptions abound. Why are psychological factors stressed? Why are patients sedated? Why are children stopped playing games rather than treated adequately? Who makes patients so scared of oral steroids?

It is to ourselves – the medical profession – we need to turn our attention. It is we who need educating about asthma and for this to be effective we need to recognize our present ignorance. This is hard to accept but its acknowledgement will save asthmatics' lives.

Delay is the other main factor found in the surveys. The failure to recognize deterioration by the patient, his relatives or the doctor can lead to fatal delay. Self-admission services such as in Edinburgh[115] can save valuable time but the local medical or geographical conditions can make this difficult to introduce. But for this to work patients must first realize how ill they are and go to hospital. Educating patients is no easy task, but for severe asthmatics to be taught to measure their peak flow on their own gauge costing only a few pounds is surely not an unattainable ideal. No general practitioner should be without his peak flow gauge. When he uses it often, patients will learn its importance by example. Its use, plus realizing the ineffectiveness of aerosol bronchodilators in a really serious attack, will promote earlier requests for help. When assistance arrives adequate treatment must be given. The odd shot of aminophylline is not enough. Overtreatment is no sin; it is undertreatment that kills. Among hospital deaths the major lapses have been in serial patient assessment. Repeat peak flows and preferably repeat arterial gases are absolutely essential. Treatment has often been passable but with many gaps. Minimum treatment for life-threatening asthma comprises oxygen (usually 35%), an intravenous infusion of 800–

2000 mg hydrocortisone per day and nebulized salbutamol/terbutaline 2.5 mg four hourly.

Education of patient and doctor is the key to preventing asthma deaths

REFERENCES

1. Scadding, J.G. (1983). Definition and clinical categories of asthma. In: Clark, T.J.H. and Godfrey, S. (eds) *Asthma*, pp. 1–11. (London: Chapman and Hall)
2. Cade, J.F. and Pain, M.C.F. (1971). Bronchial reactivity: its measurement and clinical significance. *Aust. N.Z. J. Med.*, **1**, 22–5
3. Williams, H. and McNicol, K.N . (1969). Prevalence, natural history and relationship of wheezy bronchitis and asthma in children. An epidemiological study. *Br. Med. J.*, **4**, 321–5
4. Lee, D.A., Winslow, N.R., Speight, A.N.P. and Hey, E.N. (1983). Prevalence and spectrum of asthma in childhood. *Br. Med. J.*, **286**, 1256–8
5. Balfour-Lynn, L., Tooley, M. and Godfrey, S. (1981). Relationship of exercise-induced asthma to clinical asthma in childhood. *Arch. Dis. Child.*, **56**, 450–4
6. Macdonald, J.B. and Cole, T.J. (1980). The flow-volume loop: reproducibility of air and helium-based tests in normal subjects. *Thorax*, **35**, 64–9
7. Kiviloog, J. (1973). Variability of bronchial hyperreactivity to exercise and methacholine in bronchial asthma. *Scand. J. Resp. Dis.*, **54**, 359–68
8. Speight, A.N.P., Lee, D.A. and Hey, E.N. (1983). Underdiagnosis and undertreatment of asthma in childhood. *Br. Med. J.*, **286**, 1253–6
9. Martin, A.J., McLennon, L.A., Landau, L.I. and Phelan, P.D. (1980). The natural history of asthma to adult life. *Br. Med. J.*, **280**, 1397–1400
10. Anderson, H.R., Bailey, P.A., Cooper, J.S. and Palmer, J.C. (1981). Influence of morbidity, illness label, and social, family, and health service factors on drug treatment of childhood asthma. *Lancet*, **2**, 1030–2
11. Godfrey, R.C. and Griffiths, N. (1976). The prevalence of immediate positive skin tests to *Dermatophagoides pteronyssinus* and grass pollen in schoolchildren. *Clin. Allergy*, **6**, 55–8
12. Sibbald, B., Horn, M.E.C., Brain, E.A. and Gregg, I. (1980). Genetic factors in childhood asthma. *Thorax*, **35**, 671–4
13. Sibbald, B. and Turner-Warwick, M. (1979). Factors influencing the prevalence of asthma among first-degree relatives of extrinsic and intrinsic asthmatics. *Thorax*, **34**, 332–7

14. Morrison Smith, J. (1976). The prevalence of asthma and wheezing in children. *Br. J. Dis. Chest*, **70**, 73–7
15. Peckham, C. and Butler, N. (1978). A national study of asthma in childhood. *J. Epidemiol. Community Health*, **32**, 79–85
16. Dawson, D., Horobin, G., Illsley, R. and Mitchell, R. (1969). A survey of childhood asthma in Aberdeen. *Lancet*, **1**, 827–30
17. Cullen, K.J. (1972). Climate and chest disorders in schoolchildren. *Br. Med. J.*, **4**, 65–7
18. Morrison Smith, J. (1961). Prevalence and natural history of asthma in schoolchildren. *Br. Med. J.*, **1**, 711–3
19. Graham, P.J., Rutter, M.L., Yule, W. and Pless, I.B. (1967). Childhood asthma: a psychosomatic disorder? Some epidemiological considerations. *Br. J. Prev. Soc. Med.*, **21**, 78–85
20. Williams, D.A. (1951) Social importance of allergic diseases, In: *Proceedings of First International Congress for Allergy*. pp. 42–64. (Basel: S. Karger)
21. Grant, G. (1957). Asthma among undergraduates at the University of Wales. *Acta Allergologica*, **11**, 37–44
22. Burr, M.L., St. Leger, A.S., Bevan, C. and Merrett, T.G. (1975). A community survey of asthmatic characteristics. *Thorax*, **30**, 663–8
23. D'Souza, M.F. (1979). What factors are associated with reported asthma in middle age? *Clin. Allergy*, **9**, 417–21
24. Burr, M.L., Charles, T.J., Roy, K. and Seaton, A. (1979). Asthma in the elderly: an epidemiological survey. *Br. Med. J.*, **1**, 1041–4
25. Gregg, I. Epidemiological aspects. In: Clark, T.J.H. and Godfrey, S. (eds) *Asthma*, Table 11.2 (London: Chapman and Hall)
26. Davis, J.R. (1976). Asthma and wheezy bronchitis in children. *Clin. Allergy*, **6**, 329–38
27. Horn, M.E.C. and Gregg, I. (1973). The role of viral infection and host factors in asthma and chronic bronchitis. *Chest*, **32**, (Suppl 4), 44–8
28. Leeder, S.R., Corkhill, R.T., Irwig, L.M., Holland, W.W. and Colley, J.R.T. (1976). Influence of family factors on asthma and wheezing during the first five years of life. *Br. J. Prev. Soc. Med.*, **30**, 213–8
29. Van der Lende, R. (1977). *Epidemiology of Chronic Non-specific Lung Disease (Chronic Bronchitis)*, (Assen: Van Gorcum): Text II: Tables
30. Collins, S. (1935). Age incidence of specific causes of illness. Based on records for 9000 families in 18 states visited periodically for 12 months, 1928–31. *Public Health Reports (Washington)*, **50**, 1404
31. Wilder, C.S. (1973). Prevalence of selected chronic respiratory conditions. *Vital Health Stat.*, **10**, 1–49
32. Schachter, J. (1975). Measurement of the prevalence of respiratory allergies by interview questionnaire. *J. Allergy. Clin. Immunol.*, **55**, 249–55
33. Stanhope, J.M., Rees, R.O. and Mangan, A.J. (1970). Asthma and wheeze in New Zealand adolescents. *N.Z. Med. J.*, **90**, 279–82
34. Van Niekerk, C.H., Weinberg, E.C., Shore, S.C., Heese, H. de V. and

Van Schalkwyk, D.J. (1979). Prevalence of asthma: a comparative study of urban and rural Xhosa children. *Clin. Allergy*, **9**, 319–24
35. Godfrey, R.C. (1975). Asthma and IgE levels in rural and urban communities of the Gambia. *Clin. Allergy*, **5**, 201–7
36. Viswanathan, R., Prasad, M., Thakur, A.K., Sinha, S.P., Prakash, N., Mody, R.K., Singh, T.R.B.P.N. and Prasad, S.N. (1969). Epidemiology of asthma in an urban population. A random morbidity survey. *J. Ind. Med. Assoc.*, **46**, 480–3
37. Mitsui, S. and Morio, S. (1977). Prognosis and cause of death in bronchial asthma in Japan. In: *Allergy and Clinical Immunology. Proceedings of 9th International Congress of Allergology* pp. 361–6. (Amsterdam: Excerpta Medica)
38. Mantle, J. and Pepys, J. (1974). Asthma amongst Tristan da Cunha islanders. *Clin. Allergy*, **4**, 161–70
39. Brown, P. and Gajdnsek, D.C. (1978). Acute and chronic pulmonary airways disease in Pacific island Micronesions. *Am. J. Epidemiol*, **108**, 266–73
40. Herxheimer, H. and Schaefer, O. (1974). Asthma in Canadian Eskimos. *N. Engl. J. Med.*, **291**, 1419
41. Herxheimer, H. (1964). Asthma in American Indians. *N. Engl. J. Med.*, **270**, 1128–9
42. Spears, J. (1975). The prevalence of allergic disease in young British-born schoolchildren of different ethnic origin. *J.R. Coll. Gen. Pract.*, **25**, 282–5
43. Mak, H., Johnson, P. and Abbey, H. (1982). Prevalence of asthma and health service utilisation of asthmatic children in an inner city. *J. Allergy Clin. Immunol.*, **70**, 367–72
44. Edfors-Lubs, M-L. (1971). Allergy in 7000 twin pairs. *Acta Allergologica*, **26**, 249–85
45. Hopp, R.J., Bewtra, A.K., Watt, G.D., Nair, N.M. and Townley, R.G. (1984). Genetic analysis of allergic disease in twins. *J. Allergy Clin. Immunol.*, **73**, 265–70
46. Bousley, H.A., Holtzman, M.J., Sheller, J.R. and Nader, J.A. (1981). Bronchial hyperreactivity. *Am. Rev. Resp. Dis.*, **121**, 389
47. Gerrard, J., Rao, B. and Morton, N. (1978). A genetic study of immunoglobulin E.. *Am. J. Hum. Genet.*, **30**, 46
48. Schwartz, M. (1952). Heredity in bronchial asthma.. *Acta Allergologica*, **5**, (Suppl. 2)
49. Sibbald, B., Horn, M.E.C. and Gregg, I. (1980). A family study of the genetic basis of asthma and wheezy bronchitis. *Arch. Dis. Child.*, **55**, 354–7
50. Hendrick, D.J., Davies, R.J. and D'Sousa, M.F. (1975). An analysis of skin test reactions in 656 asthmatic patients. *Thorax*, **30**, 2–8
51. Fagerberg, E. (1957). Studies in bronchial asthma II. *Acta Allergologica*, **2**, 327–42
52. Ford, R.M. (1969). Aetiology of asthma: A review of 11,551 cases (1958–1968) . *Med. J. Aust.*, **1**, 628–31
53. Horn, M.E.C. and Gregg, I. (1973). The role of viral infection and

host factors in asthma and chronic bronchitis. *Chest*, (Suppl. 4) 44–8
54. Broder, I., Higgins, M.W. and Matthews, K.P. (1974). Epidemiology of asthma and allergic rhinitis in a total community: Tecumseh, Michigan. *J. Allergy Clin. Immunol.*, **53**, 127–38
55. Smith, J.M. and Knowler, L.A. (1965). Epidemiology of asthma and allergic rhinitis. *Am. Rev. Resp. Dis.*, **92**, 16–30
56. Smith, J.M. and Knowler, L.A. (1965). Epidemiology of asthma and allergic rhinitis. *Am. Rev. Resp. Dis.*, **92**, 31–38
57. McNichol, K.N. and Williams, H.E. (1973). Spectrum of asthma in children II. Allergic components. *Br. Med. J.*, **4**, 12–16
58. Morrison Smith, J. (1983). Epidemiology and natural history of asthma, allergic rhinitis and atopic dermatitis (eczema). In: Middleton E. *et al* (eds) *Allergy: Principles and Practice* (St. Louis: C.V. Mosby)
59. Bendixen, G. (1981). The atopic state: In: Steffen, C. and Ludwig, H. (eds) *Clinical Immunology and Allergology* pp 323–30. (Amsterdam: Elsevier/North Holland Biomedical Press))
60. Frankland, A.W. (1953). Locust sensitivity. *Ann. Allergy*, **11**, 445–53
61. Kangamimori, S., Naruse, Y. and Watanebe, M. (1982). An epidemiological study on total and specific IgE levels in Japanese schoolchildren. *Clin. Allergy*, **12**, 561–8
62. Pepys, J., Parish, W.E., Stenius Aarniala, B. and Wide, L. (1979). Clinical correlations between long-term (IgE) and short-term (IgG S-TS) anaphylactic antibodies in atopic and 'non-atopic' subjects with respiratory allergic disease. *Clin. Allergy*, **9**, 645–58
63. Turner, K.J., Dowse, G.K., Stewart, G.A., Alpers, M.P. and Woolcock, A.J. (1985). Prevalence of asthma in the South Fore people of the Okapa district of Papua New Guinea. *Int. Arch. Allergy Appl. Immunol.*, **77**, 158–62
64. Macfarlane, J.T., Batchelor, M., Ridyard, J.B. and Ball, P.A.J. (1979). Asthma IgE and environment in Northern Nigeria. *Clin. Allergy*, **9**, 333–7
65. Woolcock, A.J., Colman, M.H. and Jones, M.W. (1978). Atopy and bronchial reactivity in Australian and Melanesian populations. *Clin. Allergy*, **8**, 155–64
66. British Thoracic Association comparison of atopic and non-atopic patients dying of asthma. *Br. J.. Dis. Chest*. (1987), **81**, 30–4
67. Gabriel, M., Cunnington, A.M., Allan, W.G.L., Pickering, C.A.C. and Wraith, D.G. (1982). Mite allergy in Hong Kong. *Clin. Allergy*, **12**, 157–71
68. Dowse, D.K., Turner, K.J., Stewart, G.A., Alpers, M.P. and Woolcock, A.J. (1985). The association between *Dermatophagoides* mites and the increasing prevalence of asthma in village communities within the Papua New Guinea highlands. *J. Allergy. Clin. Immunol.*, **75**, 75–83
69. Hippocrates. *Aphorisms* III 19.22
70. Khot, A., Burn, R., Evans, N., Lenney, C. and Lenney, W. (1984). Seasonal variation and time trends in childhood asthma in England and Wales 1975–81. *Br. Med. J.*, **289**, 235–7

71. Ayres, J.G. (1986). Trends in asthma and hay fever in general practice in the United Kingdom 1976–83. *Thorax*, **41**, 111–6
72. Wellivir, R.C. (1983). Upper respiratory infections in asthma. *J. Allergy Clin. Immunol.*, **72**, 341–6
73. Horn, M.E.C., Brown, E., Gregg, I., Yealland, S.J. and Inglis, J.M. (1975). Respiratory viral infections in childhood. A survey in general practice. Roehampton 1967–72. *J. Hyg.*, **74**, 157–68
74. van Bronswijk, J.E.M.H. (1973). *Dermatophagoides pteronyssinus* (Trouessant 1897) in mattress and floor dust in a temperate climate. *J. Med. Entomol.*, **10**, 63–70
75. Goldstein, I.F. (1980). Weather patterns and asthma epidemics in New York City and New Orleans. U.S.A. *Int. J. Biometeorol.*, **24**, 329–39
76. Pearson, R.S.B. (1958). Natural history of asthma. *Acta Allergologica*, **12**, 277–91
77. Zealley, A.K., Aitken, R.C.B. and Rosenthal, S.V. (1971). Personality and bronchial asthma. *Proc. Roy. Soc. Med.*, **64**, 825–9
78. Herbert, M. (1965). Personality factors and bronchial asthma: a study of South African Indian children. *J. Psychosom. Res.*, **8**, 353–64
79. Graham, P.J., Rutter, M.L., Yule, W. and Pless, I.B. (1967). Childhood asthma: A psychosomatic disorder? Some epidemiological considerations. *Br. J. Prev. Soc. Med.*, **21**, 78–85
80. Rackemann, F.M. and Edwards, M.C. (1952). Asthma in children. *N. Engl. J. Med.*, **246**, 858–63
81. Martin, A.J., McLennan, L.A., Landau, L.I. and Phelan, P.D. (1980). The natural history of childhood asthma to adult life. *Br. Med. J.*, **1**, 1397–1400
82. Martin, A.J., Landau, L.I. and Phelan, P.D. (1980). Lung function in young adults who had asthma in childhood. *Am. Rev. Resp. Dis.*, **122**, 609–16
83. Springett, V.H. (1969). Hospital admission and absence from work attributed to asthma. *Br. Med. J.*, **1**, 402–3
84. Anderson, H.R. (1978). Increase in hospitalisation for childhood asthma. *Arch. Dis. Child.*, **53**, 295–300
85. Department of Health and Social Security and Office of Population Consensus and Surveys. *Hospital Inpatient Enquiry*. Main tables 1974–83. Series M.B.H. nos. 2, 5, 7, 10, 12, 14, 16, 18, 21, 23. (London: H.M.S.O.) (1978–85)
86. Anderson, H.R., Bailey, P. and West, S. (1980). Trends in hospital care of acute childhood asthma 1970–8: a regional study. *Br. Med. J.*, **281**, 1191–4
87. Khot, A. and Burn, R. (1984). Deaths from asthma. *Br. Med. J.*, **289**, 557
88. Burney, P.G.J. (1986). Asthma mortality in England and Wales: evidence for a further increase 1974–84. *Lancet*, **2**, 323–6
89. Jackson, R.T., Beaglehole, R., Rea, H.H. and Sutherland, D.C. (1982). Mortality from asthma: a new epidemic in New Zealand. *Br. Med. J.*, **285**, 771–4
90. Sears, M.R., Rea, H.H., Beaglehole, R. *et al.* (1985). Asthma mortality in New Zealand: a two-year national study. *N.Z. Med. J.*, **98**, 271–5

91. Sly, R.M. (1984). Increases in deaths from asthma. *Ann. Allergy*, **53**, 20–5
92. Fleming, D.M. and Crombie, D.L. (1987). Prevalence of asthma and hay fever in England and Wales. *Br. Med. J.*, **294**, 279–83
93. A subcommittee of the BTA Research Committee. Accuracy of death certificates in bronchial asthma. *Thorax*, (1984), **39**, 505–9
94. Ormerod, L.P. and Stableforth, D.E. (1980). Asthma mortality in Birmingham 1975–7: 53 deaths. *Br. Med. J.*, **280**, 687–90
95. Macdonald, J.B., Seaton, A. and Williams, D.A. (1976). Asthma deaths in Cardiff 1963–74: 90 deaths outside hospital. *Br. Med. J.*, **1**, 1493–5
96. Macdonald, J.B., Macdonald, E.T., Seaton A. and Williams, D.A. (1976). Asthma deaths in Cardiff 1963–74: 53 deaths in hospital. *Br. Med. J.*, **2**, 721–3
97. Johnson, A.J., Nunn, A.J., Somner, A.R., Stableforth, D.E. and Stewart, D.J. (1984). Circumstances of death from asthma. *Br. Med. J.*, **288**, 1870–2
98. Sears, M.R., Rea, H.H., Fenwick, J., Gillies, A.J.D., Holst, P.E., O'Donnell, T.V. and Rothwell, R.P.G. (1987). 75 deaths in asthmatics prescribed home nebulizers. *Br. Med. J.*, **294**, 477–80
99. Khot, A. and Burn, R. (1984). Seasonal variation and time trends of deaths from asthma in England and Wales 1960–82. *Br. Med. J.*, **289**, 233–4
100. Johnson, A.J., Nunn, A.J., Somner, A.R., Stableforth, D.E. and Stewart, C.S. (1984). Circumstances of death from asthma. *Br. Med. J.*, **288**, 1870–2
101. Keating, G., Mitchell, E.A., Jackson, R., Beaglehole, R. and Rea, H. (1984). Trends in the sales of drugs for asthma in New Zealand, Australia, and the United Kingdom, 1975–81. *Br. Med. J.*, **289**, 348–351
102. Macdonald, E.T. and Macdonald, J.B. (1982). *Drug Treatment in the Elderly*. pp 195–239 (Chichester: John Wiley and Sons)
103. Speizer, F.E., Doll, R., Heaf, P. and Strang, L.B. (1968). Investigation into the use of drugs preceding death from asthma. *Br. Med. J.*, **1**, 339–343
104. Fraser, P.M., Speizer, F.E., Waters, S.D.M., Doll, R. and Mann, N.M. (1971). The circumstances preceding death from asthma in young people in 1968 to 1969. *Br. J. Dis. Chest*, **65**, 71–84
105. Arnold, A.G., Lane, D.J. and Zapata, E. (1982). The speed of onset and severity of acute severe asthma. *Br. J. Dis. Chest*, **76**, 157–63
106. Rubinfield, A.R. and Pain, M.C.F. (1976). Perception of asthma. *Lancet*, **1**, 882–7
107. Burdon, J.P.W., Juniper, E.F., Killian, K.J., Hargreave, F.E. and Campbell, E.J.M. (1982). The perception of breathlessness in asthma. *Am. Rev. Resp. Dis.*, **126**, 825–8
108. Ganderia, B. (1973). Pressurised sympathomimetic aerosols and their lack of relationship to asthma mortality in Australia. *Med. J. Aust.*, **1**, 273–7

109. Stolley, P.D. and Schinner, R. (1978). Association between asthma, mortality and isoproterenol inhalers: a review. *Prev. Med.*, **7**, 519–38
110. Sears, M.R., Rea, H.H., Rothwell, R.P.G. *et al.* (1986). Asthma mortality: comparison between New Zealand and England. *Br. Med. J.*, **293**, 1342–5
111. Wilson, J.D., Sutherland, D.C. and Thomas, A.K. (1981). Has the change to beta-agonists combined with oral theophyllines increased cases of fatal asthma? *Lancet*, **1**, 1235–7
112. Grant, I.W.B. (1981). Has the change to beta-agonists combined with oral theophyllines increased cases of fatal asthma? *Lancet*, **2**, 36–7
113. Grant, I.W.B. (1983). Asthma in New Zealand. *Br. Med. J.*, **286**, 374–7
114. Seaton, A. (1978). Asthma – contrasts in care. *Thorax*, **33**, 1–2
115. Crompton, G.K., Grant, I.W.B. and Bloomfield, P. (1979). Edinburgh emergency asthma admission service: report on 10 years' experience. *Br. Med. J.*, **4**, 1199–201
116. Hill, A.E. (1966). Asthma among schoolchildren. *J. School Health*, **36**, 353–6
117. Partridge, M.R., Gibson, G.J. and Pride, N.B. (1979). Asthma in Asian immigrants. *Clin. Allergy*, **9**, 489–94
118. Stewart, C.J. and Nunn, A.J. (1985). Are asthma mortality rates rising? *Br. J. Dis. Chest*, **79**, 229–34

3

PHYSIOLOGY AND CLINICAL PATHOLOGY OF ASTHMA

Introduction

Traditional definitions of asthma have been almost totally empirical and descriptive and dependent upon recognizing intermittent and reversible airflow obstruction. For example, the Ciba Symposium of 1959 defined the condition in these terms: '... widespread narrowing of the bronchial airways, which changes its severity over short periods of time, either spontaneously or under treatment, and is not due to cardiovascular disease'. This is still widely quoted, and forms the basis of most of our diagnostic judgements. Most clinicians would probably accept a spontaneous or induced change of about 15% in peak expiratory flow rate (PEFR) or the forced expiratory volume in one second (FEV_1) as being sufficiently great to warrant the diagnosis (Fig. 3.1).

The patient, of course, will give a history of intermittent wheeze, irritant cough, chest tightness and dyspnoea, but if given a peak flow meter to carry around and have at home will be able to demonstrate that the symptoms correspond to dips in the PEFR (Fig. 3.2). Other smaller but frequently

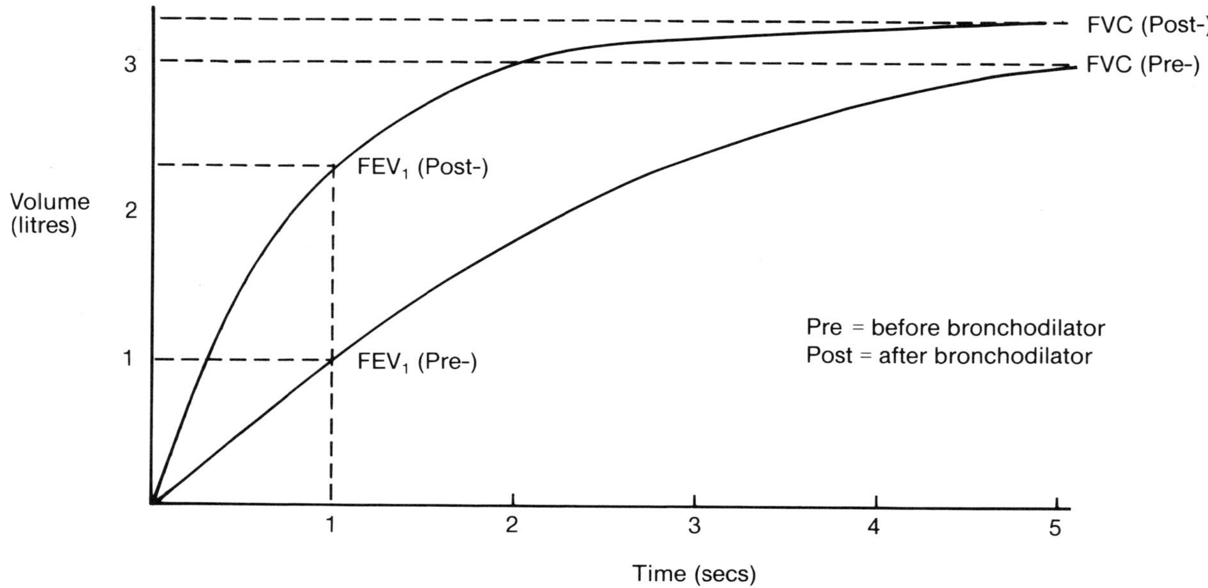

Figure 3.1 Bronchodilator-induced changes in the spirogram in an asthmatic

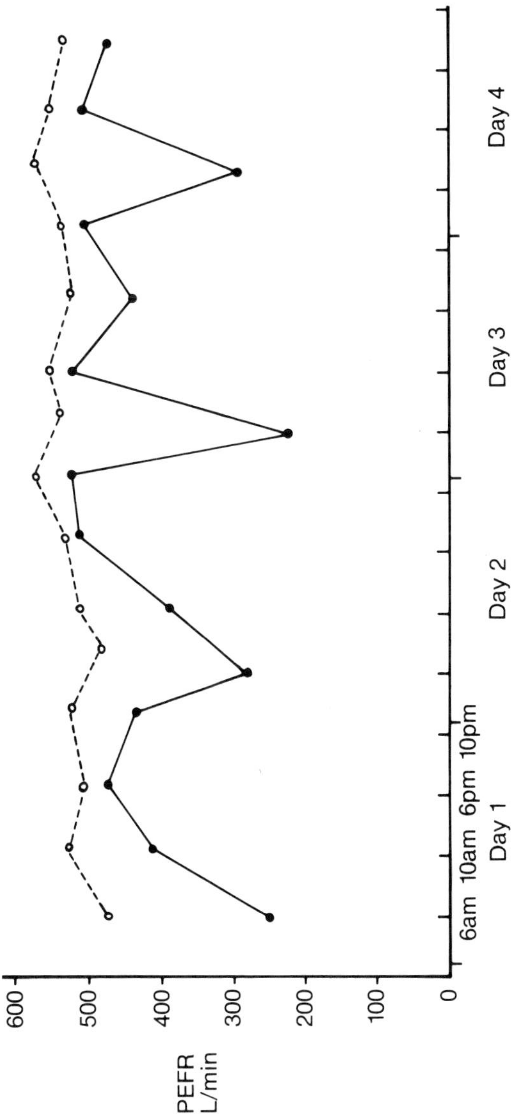

●——● trace obtained before treatment, with marked variation in PEFR, with dramatic 'dips' especially first thing in the morning

o- - -o trace obtained after a period of 'prophylactic' therapy with corticosteroids

Figure 3.2 Peak expiratory flow chart in an asthmatic

significant dips in PEFR will also occur even when the patient is essentially asymptomatic. Thus, both the patient and the physician recognize the disease in terms of related clinical and physiological phenomena. Certain temporal relationships are similarly recognized empirically as being important, e.g. symptoms and dips in air flow at night or first thing in the morning; on exercise, particularly in cold, dry air; or on exposure to smokey or foggy atmospheres[1].

From the purely pragmatic perspective, therefore, it could be argued that there is little more to asthma, at least in terms of making a diagnosis, than taking a good respiratory history and organizing some basic physiological monitoring of airflow. The success of this pragmatic approach, however, had tended to obscure the sad reality of a profound lack of understanding about the pathophysiological processes underlying these empirical phenomena that both doctors and patients observe. Until remarkably recently there has also been an equally lamentable paucity of basic research aimed at trying to unravel some of these mysteries. Most research has been directed towards defining the multitude of physical or chemical stimuli that will cause the airways to constrict, and in developing smooth muscle relaxants which will reverse the muscle contraction.

THE CONCEPT OF AIRWAY HYPER-RESPONSIVENESS IN ASTHMA

A fundamental property of the airways in active asthma is a tendency to acutely narrow, due to airway smooth muscle contraction, at a level of bronchoconstrictor stimulus that would not affect normal airways. This characteristic property of asthmatic airways has been variously referred to as bronchial hyper-reactivity', 'bronchial hyper-excitability' or 'bronchial hyper-irritability'[2]. The term airway hyper-responsiveness has come to largely replace these earlier terms because it is more descriptive and avoids possible mechanistic connotations. Further, the term 'reactivity' has also taken on a more specific meaning in some literature, being used for the 'rate' of narrowing of stimulated airways[3].

Airway hyper-responsiveness can be demonstrated with so called 'non-specific stimuli' such as exercise, isocapnic hyperventilation (particularly with cold, dry air), or osmotic challenge to the airways with a water aerosol or alternatively with an aerosolized hyperosmolar salt solution[1]. These qualitative and essentially single dose challenges have been largely replaced, at least in the laboratory setting, by a more quantitative approach with the use of specific contractile agonists such as methacholine or histamine, which are usually given by inhalation in sequential incremental doses at fixed time intervals until a set level of bronchoconstriction has been achieved. The index of airway calibre most frequently used in such studies has been the FEV_1 and the dose of agonist causing precisely a 20% fall in FEV_1 has most frequently been the value taken and is read off by direct linear interpolation from a plotted dose-response curve (Fig. 3.3). The dose is usually plotted on a logarithmic scale, as in more classical pharmacological studies. The value thus obtained from such a study is called by convention the PD_{20} FEV_1 (the provocation dose causing a 20% fall in FEV_1). This has become the international 'unit of currency' in the field of airway responsiveness, and eventually may become as familiar in general use as conventional spirometric values are at present.

A minority of workers have used specific airway conductance (sGaw) [measured in a body plethysmograph], or maximum flow at 25% or 40% of vital capacity (V_{25} or V_{40}) [from partial flow–volume curves] as the index of airway narrowing in measurement of indices of airway responsiveness. Although more sensitive and allowing an earlier and greater change in airway diameter to be demonstrated, these are also more difficult and less reproducible measurements to make, and are probably best thought of still as research tools for pharmacological experiments.

There are, in general, two techniques for delivering agonist

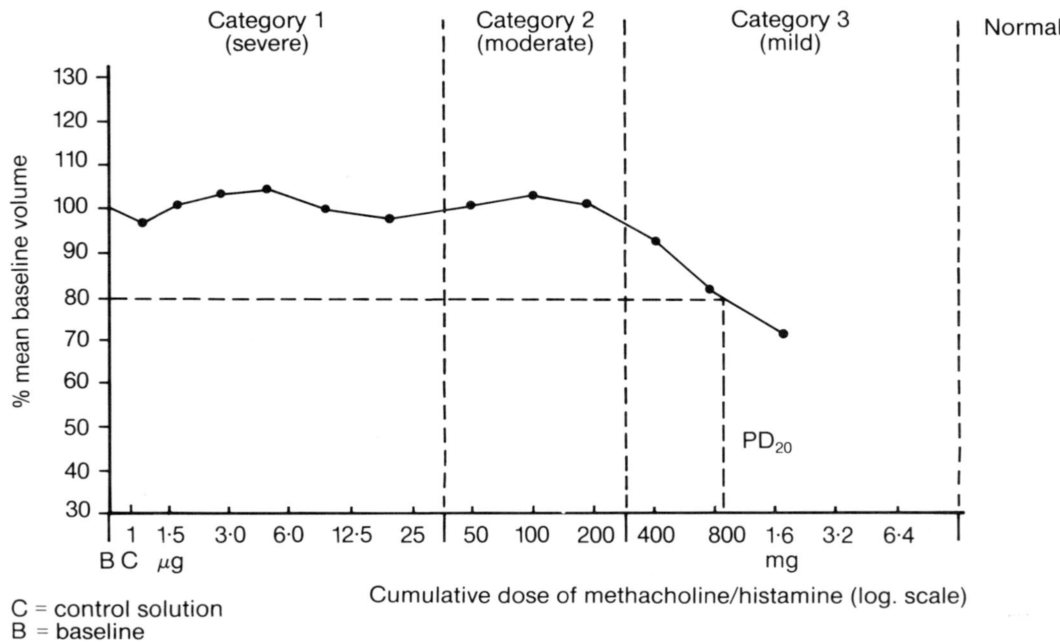

Figure 3.3 Measurement of PD_{20} FEV_1 by histamine or methacholine challenge (Newcastle General Hospital)

drugs to the airways in bronchoconstrictor challenges for measurement of PD_{20}. The most widely used is the 'tidal breathing' method popularized by the McMaster University group in Canada, which uses a jet nebulizer to continuously generate an aerosol of the drug which is inhaled via a face mask or mouth piece during normal tidal breathing over 2 min. The doses are repeated at 5 min intervals by increasing the concentration of drug in the nebulizer chamber, and FEV_1 is measured before each repeated dose[4]. The alternative 'dosimeter' method, which has the endorsement of professional bodies on both sides of the Atlantic, attempts to control as precisely as possible the actual dose of drug delivered to the airways[5]. In Newcastle, we have developed such a device which uses a microprocessor to control a breath activated nebulizer which then generates aerosol for exactly 2 s. The system delivers to the airways 10 μl of drug solution ($\pm 5\%$) per activation. Five inhalations are taken at 5 min intervals with doubling concentrations of either histamine or methacholine. This method allows a more rapid measurement of PD_{20} but also requires very much more expensive equipment.

In the best of hands the tidal breathing method is highly reproducible, with the McMaster group achieving 95% confidence limits for repeat measurements of PD_{20} FEV_1 in asthmatics of less than 1.5 doubling doses$_6$. However, results have been much more variable in other hands[7,8]. The Newcastle dosimeter system has achieved an accuracy marginally better than that achieved by Hargreaves *et al.*, with a 95% confidence interval for repeat PD_{20} measurements in stable asthmatics over a short period of time of less than 1 doubling dose for both methacholine and histamine. For widespread use the tidal breathing method probably still provides better value for money, but every attention must be paid to accuracy of measurement, and one should not be satisfied with a reproducibility much worse than one halving or doubling in PD_{20} FEV_1.

THE CLINICAL RELEVANCE OF AIRWAY HYPER-RESPONSIVENESS

Fig. 3.4 illustrates a series of dose-response curves to histamine in 30 relatively mild asthmatics (three left hand panels) compared to 30 normal, non-asthmatic, non-atopic controls (three right hand panels). The response to histamine was measured in terms of sGaw, and the dose of histamine plotted cumulatively. It can be seen that the range of concentrations of drug needed to obtain a 20% fall in sGaw in the asthmatics ranged from approximately 0.1 mg/ml to 1 mg/ml while in the normals it ran from about 2 mg/ml to 20 mg/ml. Thus, in this group of subjects the difference in responsiveness between the asthmatics and the normal group was little more than a single log. shift in histamine concentrations – relatively little by classic pharmacological standards. Furthermore, there was hardly any difference in histamine response characteristics between the least responsive asthmatics and the most responsive normals.

In these terms, therefore, the difference between someone labelled an asthmatic and a normal subject can hardly be regarded as all or none, but rather as a spectrum which merges at one end into the normal range.

Whether a subject at any given point in the spectrum of responsiveness develops bronchoconstriction and therefore symptoms, will depend upon the balance between their level of responsiveness and the level of airway muscle contractile stimulus to which they are exposed. Thus, a person with a relatively low degree of airway responsiveness (high value for PD_{20}) will require an intense stimulus before symptomatic bronchoconstriction ensues, while in someone with a high degree of bronchial responsiveness a relatively trivial stimulus, which would not normally cause bronchoconstriction, may have major effects upon the airways (Fig 3.5). Many studies have demonstrated the clinical significance of an individual's level of airway hyper-responsiveness. Thus the severity of clinical asthma and the need for anti-asthma treatments[8], the

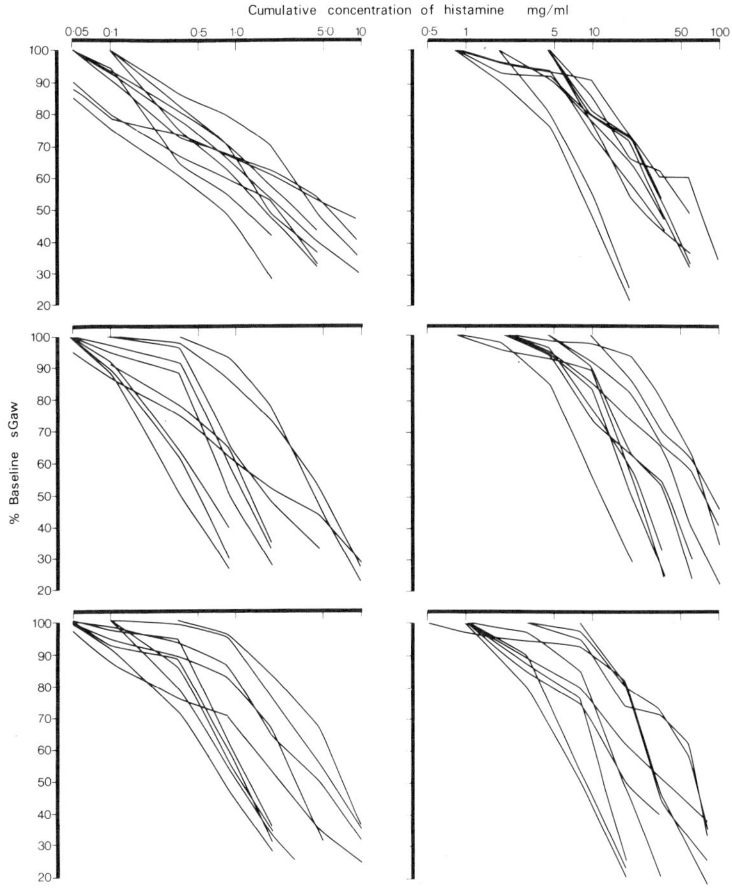

Figure 3.4 Comparison of inhalation histamine dose-response curves in asthmatic (left panels, $n=30$) and normal (right panels, $n=30$) individuals

degree of diurnal variation in PEFR and the susceptibility to non-specific stimuli such as exercise[9], can all be directly related to the PD_{20} methacholine or histamine within an asthmatic population. Perhaps, therefore, the disease we call asthma could better be regarded as '*symptomatic airway hyper-responsiveness*'.

The extent of 'fixed', inherent and presumably genetically-determined hyper-responsiveness in the community at large is

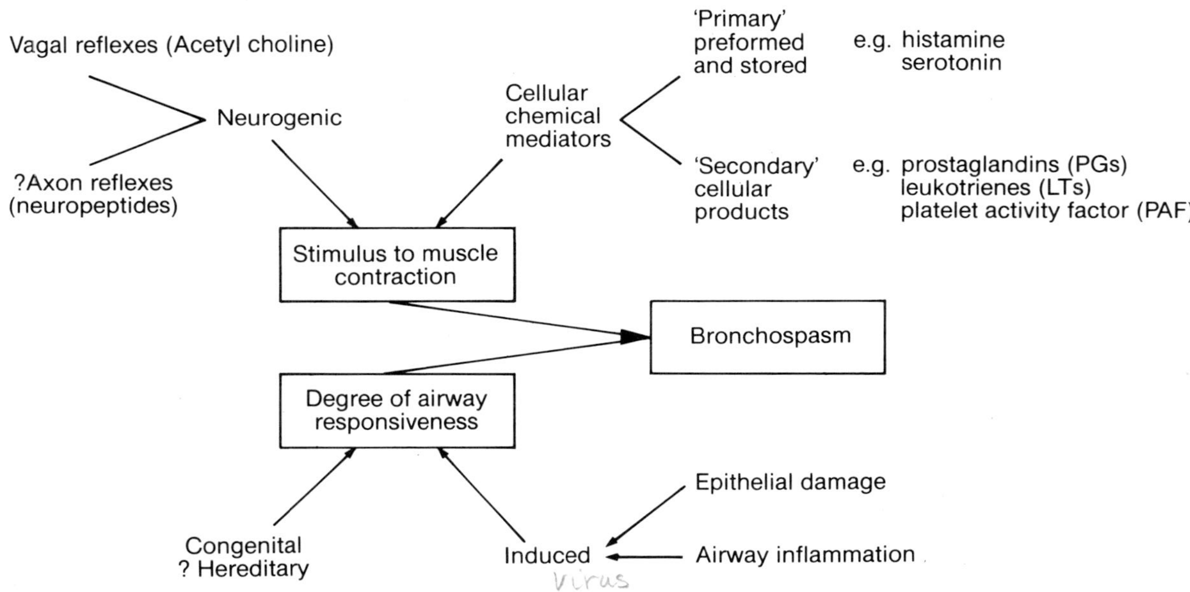

Figure 3.5 Bronchoconstriction is the product of a balance between the stimulus to airway smooth muscle contraction and the degree of responsiveness of the muscle to the stimulus. When the airways are relatively unresponsive, the stimulus to contraction has to be large to induce bronchospasm. but the same degree of airway narrowing will occur with a much smaller stimulus if the airways are hyper-responsive

not yet well defined, but is probably an important component of the asthmatic problem that we have to deal with[10]. Perhaps of even greater importance, however, certainly from the therapeutic point of view, and also in terms of understanding the underlying disease process in perhaps the majority of patients, is the fascinating fact that hyper-responsiveness can be induced *de novo* in an individual, or can be further increased significantly in an individual with an already measurable degree of airway hyper-responsiveness[11].

The list of such 'inducers' of airway hyper-responsiveness is quite substantial and includes:

viral infection of the respiratory tract[12];
antigen exposure in sensitized individual[13];
ozone[14];
oxides of nitrogen[15]; and
industrial sensitizers, e.g. isocyanates, epoxyresins, formaldehyde, wood dusts[16].

Thus, the degree of airway (smooth muscle) responsiveness is of pivotal importance in asthma, and this realization is essential for an understanding of what everyday asthma is actually about. It may also be of great potential relevance for the present and future management of individual patients. We know that there are many different potential physical and environmental stimuli to airway narrowing, and a wide variety of potential chemical mediators of muscle contraction available within the airway mucosa, all of which could be released under the right circumstances. Such locally available cellularly-generated contractile agents include histamine, serotonin, prostaglandins (PGs), thromboxane (Tx), sulphidopeptide leukotrienes (LTs) (formerly known as slow reacting substance of anaphylaxis or SRS-A), platelet activating factor (PAF), and various peptides and tachykinins[11]. In addition, acetylcholine can also be released from cholinergic nerve endings by vagal reflex stimulation[17]. With so many contractile influences at work it is not surprising that most research directed at trying to find *specific* antagonists of bronchoconstriction have largely failed to impress, because if only one agonist is countered, there are still many more continuing to be active. Thus we have come to rely therapeutically on broad physiological antagonists of bronchoconstriction, however induced, such as the bronchodilator sympathomimetics and the theophyllines. If, however, one could discover the key to the modulation of airway responsiveness and *specifically* antagonize the agent responsible, then one really would have the prospect of a fundamental improvement in asthma therapy.

AIRWAY INFLAMMATION IN ASTHMA

The classical description of acute inflammation, rather like the classical description of asthma, was empirical and was based upon the observation of:

(1) redness, because of vasodilatation;
(2) oedema, because of vascular permeability; and
(3) pain, because of local stimulation of nerve endings.

When the inflammatory process involved a mucous membrane it was also observed that there was hypersecretion from mucous glands and desquamation of epithelial cells[18]. Modern understanding of inflammation, although still incomplete, includes insights into a much more complex reaction involving the accumulation and activation of a variety of cell types, e.g. neutrophils, eosinophils, macrophages, and lymphocytes with the local production of a variety of mediators – some from cellular stores and others newly generated, which cause the vascular and permeability changes, stimulate pain fibres, and in addition bring about a variable degree of local damage. Within this framework of 'militant chaos', factors, again poorly understood, must be invoked which limit the inflammatory response and lead either to healing of the tissue or the stimulation of fibrocytic cells which lay down collagen causing scarring. To complicate the situation further, it is evident that the various potential components of the inflammatory response are not necessarily all recruited, or at least not to the same extent in every situation nor at the same stage in the evolution of the process.

It has been known for many years that many features of classical inflammation are present in the airway wall of patients dying of asthma[19]. We also know that patients with acute asthma frequently cough up thick mucus plugs containing inflammatory cells and epithelial debris as well as Charcot–Leyden crystals and Curshmann's spirals of glycoprotein. Traditionally, the potential importance of these inflammatory changes was thought to lie predominantly in causing at least some of the severe and relatively refractory narrowing of the airways that occurs in acute severe asthma, by a mixture of mucus plugging and airway swelling. The actual mechanical importance of these changes is still poorly defined. However, it is now realized from data obtained in a limited number of studies in which the airway wall has been biopsied[20] or the airway lumen washed out (lavaged) via a bronchoscope[21], that changes compatible with an inflammatory process are also present in the airways even in relatively stable and well asthmatics. These findings include widespread epithelial cellular damage and desquamation, and infiltration of the airways with neutrophils and eosinophils.

RELATIONSHIPS BETWEEN AIRWAY HYPER-RESPONSIVENESS AND AIRWAY INFLAMMATION

Most, if not all, of the factors listed above as potential inducers of airway hyper-responsiveness, e.g. infection, allergen challenge, ozone and reactive chemicals in industry, could be expected, at least hypothetically, to lead to both acute injury of the airway lining, and also to a subsequent acute inflammatory reaction. This potential, linked to the observations that there may indeed be an ongoing acute inflammatory reaction in the airways in asthmatics has lead to the concept that inflammation, or at least some final common 'influence' within the inflammatory milieu is responsible for 'turning on' the airway smooth muscle to become hyper-responsive. Most of the evidence available to support this theory has come from animal studies, but there is now an increasing amount of data from human studies also to back up the idea that bronchial asthma, or at least 'symptomatic airway hyper-responsiveness' may in fact be caused, at a pathophysiological level, by 'inflammatory airway disease', however that is initiated. For the first time this gives a broad-based pathological correlation to this common disease that we see in clinical practice.

Evidence from animal studies

Several groups of workers over recent years have carried out experiments in various species of animal in which the airways have been made hyper-responsive by challenge with a 'sensitizing' agent, and the subsequent pathological changes in the airways monitored. The first and most comprehensive series of such studies was performed by Professor J. A. Nadel's group at the Cardiovascular Research Institute in San Francisco, using a model in which airway hyper-responsiveness was induced by exposing the animals to an atmosphere containing up to 3 ppm of ozone for 2 h[22]. Ozone was chosen as it is a significant atmospheric pollutant in sunny West Coast US cities and has been described as a cause of hyper-responsiveness and worsening asthma in man[23]. In dogs exposed to 2 ppm of ozone increased airway responses to inhaled acetylcholine was demonstrated in approximately 50% of animals at 1 h after leaving the exposure chamber. Large airway biopsies were obtained at the same time via a rigid bronchoscope and were found to contain a large influx of polymorphonuclear neutrophil leukocytes *only* in those animals that had become hyper-responsive[24]. Furthermore, there was a close correlation between the increase in response to acetylcholine obtained and the increase in neutrophil count in the airway biopsies (compared to a control run)[24]. Thus for the first time there was direct evidence of at least an association between the induction of airway responsiveness and the provocation of an acute inflammatory response. Airway washings also showed a high neutrophilia and also a large increase in desquamated epithelial cells in the airways at the time of increase in bronchoconstrictor responsiveness, suggesting that the airway epithelium had been damaged[25]. Stimulation of airway epithelial cells from the dog *in vitro* was shown to cause release of leukotriene B_4 (LTB_4) a potent chemotactic agent from neutrophils[26], and indeed in the biopsies there was a gradient of neutrophils from the mucosal blood vessels out to the airway lumen, suggestive of active recruitment of cells.

In subsequent experiments using the same model, hydroxyurea was used to deplete the animals fairly specifically of neutrophils and this was found to prevent the ozone-induced increase in responsiveness and the airway neutrophilia, although the epithelial damage still occurred[27]. Indomethacin, a potent inhibitor of prostaglandin and thromboxane production, also inhibited the change in responsiveness after ozone, but *without* preventing either the airway damage *or* the airway neutrophilia[28]. Thus, the strategic effector cell in this sequence of events was very suggestively the neutrophil while the chemical inducer of the responsiveness change was apparently one of the prostaglandin family. In subsequent experiments, airway washings in ozone-exposed dogs were found to contain a high concentration of thromboxane B_2 (TxB_2), a metabolite of TxA_2, and indeed inhalation of freshly generated TxA_2 induced hyper-responsiveness[29]. The hyper-responsive change after ozone could be blocked by a specific thromboxane synthesis inhibitor[30]. Thus, in this specific example of an animal model of induced airway hyper-responsiveness which has been worked out in some detail, it would seem that the arachidonic acid metabolite TxA_2 is specifically responsible for the pharmacological changes demonstrable, although the influx of neutrophils is essential, either to directly produce the Tx or to stimulate its production by some other local cell type (Fig. 3.6).

Similar but as yet less conclusive findings have also been reported in both a sensitized rabbit and dog model using antigen as the inducer of hyper-responsiveness[31].

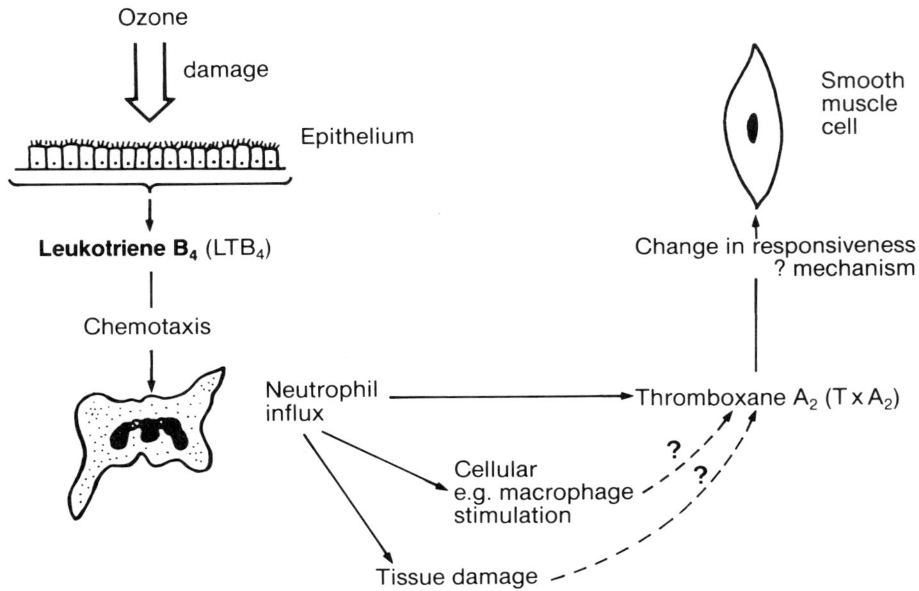

Figure 3.6 An outline of the mechanisms involved in ozone-induced airway hyper-responsiveness in dogs

However, in other systems the mechanism is much less clear cut. In the guinea pig both ozone and cigarette smoke have been used to induce a state of hyper-responsiveness[32,33], but in neither situation does this seem related to cellular influx, but rather to a direct disruption of the mucosal epithelial tight-junctions and possibly to the production of leukotrienes. On the other hand, when toluene di-isocyanate was used as the inducer of the airway change in the guinea pig, a neutrophil influx did seem to be an important factor[34].

Evidence in humans

Pathological and cellular studies

Inevitably, accumulation of evidence for a direct link between airway hyper-responsiveness and airway inflammation in humans has been slow. The original observations of inflammation in the airways of asthmatic patients at post-mortem examination[19], as well as more recent limited biopsy[20] and bronchoalveolar lavage[21] data in humans, have already been mentioned. These studies have all been consistent with at least a low grade inflammatory reaction in the airways of even stable asthmatics, with a much more intense response in the acutely ill.

In terms of the cell types involved in the inflammatory process the *eosinophil* has been mentioned most prominently in most studies, rather than the neutrophil, and indeed we are all familiar with the examination of sputum for eosinophils as a frequent part of the preliminary work-up of suspected asthmatics. Recently, De Monchy *et al.*[35] reported a pre-dominant eosinophilia in the airways of asthmatics at lavage during the late reaction after an antigen challenge. There was also an increase in lavage fluid concentration of eosinophilic cationic protein, indicative of an increase in eosinophil degranulation within the airways. A relationship has been reported between the degree of airway responsiveness in asthmatics and the numbers of circulatory eosinophils in the blood[36].

In contrast to this emphasis on the eosinophil as the cell of note in asthmatic airways, there are now a number of important studies which have highlighted the potential aetiological involvement of the *neutrophil* in human asthmatic hyper-responsiveness. Thus exposure of human subjects to ozone (0.4–0.6 ppm) not only caused an increase in the broncho-constrictor response to methacholine, but also induced an associated neutrophil influx into bronchoalveolar lavage fluid[37]. An intense neutrophil cellular response has also been reported in the airways in association with the hyper-responsiveness induced by toluene di-isocyanate challenge in sensitized workers[38]. Finally, in a study in Newcastle over the past 18 months, over 20 stable patients with asthma have undergone fibreoptic bronchoscopy and bronchoalveolar lavage of a middle lobe segment. Differential cell counts have shown an increase in both neutrophils and eosinophils in asthmatic airways compared to normal controls, but only the percentage neutrophil count, and not the eosinophil count, correlated significantly with pre-measured airway responsiveness to methacholine.

Of course, neither the neutrophil nor the eosinophil, separately or together, would exhaust the possibilities for cellular involvement in asthma-related airway inflammation. In the Newcastle study just mentioned, there was a slight but non-significant increase in the total numbers of *macrophages* present in the asthmatic lavages, but even more interestingly the degree of measured macrophage cellular activity was greatly increased above normal in asthmatics.

The *mast cell*, although forming a very small percentage of airway cells, has long been thought of as a predominant cell in asthma. Although general enthusiasm for the pre-eminent importance of the mast cell has greatly waned over recent years, the small number of intraluminal mast cells, which are capable of releasing a wide variety of contractile and inflammatory mediators and chemotactic chemicals, is very strategically placed to initiate many of the acute events occurring after a variety of different airway challenges. Although still a very small percentage of the total cell population the numbers of mast cells are increased in bronchoalveolar lavage fluid from asthmatics[39], and the numbers of mast cells present have been reported to correlate with airway hyper-responsiveness in atopic asthmatics (P. M. O'Byrne, pers. commun.).

A more recent addition to the list of cells which were traditionally included in those thought of as likely contributors to an acute inflammatory response is the *platelet*. After antigen challenge in sensitized human asthmatics, platelets have been recovered in lavage fluid[40] and have been found to be activated within the circulation[41]. Platelets, like macrophages, and in addition to the more classically accepted mast cells, can be activated by antigen through an IgE-dependent mechanism[42].

Mediator studies

A major stimulus to interest in the possibility that inflammation in the airways may be important for the induction of a hyper-responsive state was the finding that normal, non-asthmatic, non-atopic volunteer subjects could be made relatively hyper-responsive to histamine by inhaling a small dose of prostaglandin $F_{2\alpha}$($PGF_{2\alpha}$) which in itself was insufficient to cause bronchoconstriction[43]. This result has been confirmed for $PGF_{2\alpha}$ by other workers, and repeated also for PGD_2[44] and also PGE_2[45]. The latter is of particular interest in some ways, and is rather paradoxical in that PGE_2 is usually thought of as a bronchodilator and smooth muscle relaxant, and yet it was found that after the bronchodilator effects of an inhaled dose had worn off, there was a period of hyper-responsiveness demonstrable.

It is probable that on the airway smooth muscle surface there is just *one* PG contractile receptor, specific for TxA_2, but shared by other PGs (including PGE_2, although its predominant effect is via a separate relaxant receptor). Thus, although this hypothesis has not yet been tested, it is likely that the induction of hyper-responsiveness by inhaled contractile PGs is mediated via the thromboxane receptor.

Inhalation of PAF, too, has been shown to induce a hyper-responsive state in a variety of animal species and also in man[46]. At least in the dog, this effect seems to be produced via stimulation of thromboxane by inflammatory cells[47].

There is very little data available on the presence of arachidonic acid metabolites or other lipid mediators in bronchoalveolar lavage fluid from asthmatics. In human volunteers made hyper-responsive by ozone challenge a large increase was found in PGE_2 and $PGF_{2\alpha}$ with a lesser increase in Tx, and no increase in leukotrienes in airway fluid[37]. A recent report from Professor Kay's group at the Brompton Hospital (*Thorax*, in press) found an increase in leukotrienes in bronchoalveolar lavage fluid from symptomatic asthmatics compared to controls. In a retrospective analysis of bronchoalveolar lavage fluid obtained from asthmatics in Newcastle, however, we have failed to find an increase in either leukotrienes or prostaglandins in stable but hyper-responsive asthmatics, although we have detected the presence of PAF in fluid from several asthmatics but not controls.

In a recent American study, elevated amounts of tissue kallikrein and kinin were found in bronchoalveolar lavage from asthmatics, and such substances too may contribute to the inflammatory oedema and bronchospasm in asthma, as well as stimulating release and production of both formed (e.g. histamine) and secondary (PGs, LTs, PAF) mediators from inflammatory cells[48]. Bradykinin may be formed by the action of a mast cell derived kininogenase and have its predominant effect by stimulating afferent C fibres exposed in the damaged airway epithelium. It has been proposed that this in turn leads to the activation of local axon reflexes and release of neuropeptides from vagal nerve endings which cause further disruption of the epithelium, mucosal oedema and chemotaxis of inflammatory cells[49]. This system would seem to be potentially a very effective way of amplifying the inflammatory response within the airways once initiated.

The effect of drugs

If a specific inflammatory mediator(s) is important for 'turning the airways on' to become hyper-responsive, then anti-inflammatory agents would be expected to be effective in preventing or reversing the induction of hyper-responsiveness. Perhaps surprisingly, there are relatively few studies which have addressed this very important question, and it is far from being conclusively answered. However, corticosteroids, although having a variety of actions, probably have as an important role in asthma the induction of an intracellular protein, macrocortin, which switches off the membrane enzyme phospholipase A_2 which cleaves arachidonic acid out of membrane phospholipids with the subsequent production of a wide range of inflammatory mediators (Fig. 3.7).

Non-steroidal anti-inflammatory drugs have not been thoroughly studied therapeutically in asthma, largely one presumes because of worries about the acute bronchoconstriction that they can induce (for as yet still poorly-defined reasons) in about 10% of patients. However, indomethacin, a potent inhibitor of the cyclooxygenase enzyme of prostaglandin synthesis has been reported to reduce airway hyper-responsiveness in asthmatics[50] and to inhibit the induction of hyper-responsiveness after immunization with live attenuated influenza virus[51], and more recently after antigen challenge (P. M. O'Byrne, pers. commun.). In a recent report a Japanese group has demonstrated a highly significant decrease in airway responsiveness in asthmatics after treatment with a specific thromboxane synthetase inhibitor, OKY-046[52].

Summary

Thus, there is increasing evidence that even in human disease the induction of a hyper-responsive state in the airways is aetiologically associated with some component of an inflammatory process within the airways. The evidence to date points to one of the prostaglandin family as being especially import-

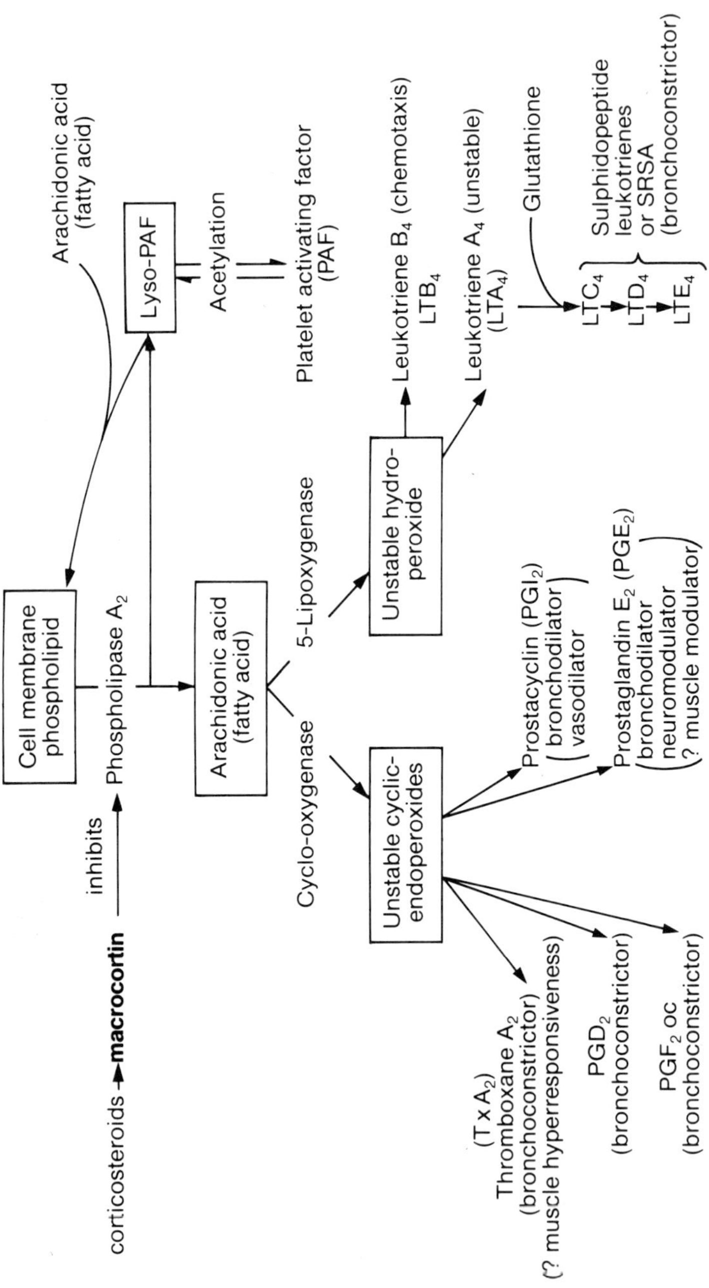

Figure 3.7 The generation of 'secondary' membrane-derived mediators

ant in this regard and the front runner for suspicion at this time is thromboxane A_2, or other contractile PGs operating through the same receptor. This raises the exciting prospect of eventually having the ability to therapeutically modulate the degree of airway responsiveness with *specific* drugs in a way that is not practicable for bronchospasm as such.

WHAT IS THE CHANGE THAT OCCURS IN HYPER-RESPONSIVE AIRWAYS?

This question has not yet been answered, but the change is presumed to be at the level of airways smooth muscle itself, since the phenomenon of hyper-responsiveness seems to be demonstrable with a wide variety of smooth muscle contractile agents in vivo[2]. Direct potentiation of airway smooth muscle constriction *in vitro* has been reported with pre-treatment with inflammatory mediators[53]. It is unlikely that such a change occurs specifically at receptor level, but is probably due to a less specific change such as calcium handling by the muscle fibres.

However, several studies have now attempted to correlate the degree of hyper-responsiveness *in vivo* in humans, with the *in vitro* responses of airway muscle subsequently obtained at thoracotomy for lung cancer[54,55]. All of these studies have *failed* to demonstrate a relationship between the two, but have been based upon recruitment of patients who were largely hyper-responsive bronchitics rather than true-bill asthmatics.

In dogs made acutely hyper-responsive to ozone and then killed[56], the airway muscle again proved to be no more responsive *in vitro* than controls. However, there was a change in the response to stimulation of postganglionic cholinergic vagal nerve endings, suggesting an increase in neurogenic release of acetylcholine. The cholinergic nerve ending has been shown to be under very sensitive prostaglandin control[57] and can be made more responsive to stimulation by thromboxane A_2[58]. However, the importance *in vivo* of such findings is somewhat doubtful because of the apparent lack of effect of anticholinergic drugs in reversing or preventing the hyper-responsive state[59].

Airway epithelium itself has been demonstrated to produce a smooth muscle relaxant agent that has not yet been defined[60]. It is possible that damage to the epithelium, that is such a prominent part of the inflammatory process in the airways, causes a depletion of this relaxant substance and that hyper-responsiveness is not due to a change in the muscle *per se*, as suggested above, but rather is caused by a fault in this normal epithelial control mechanism.

PROVOCATION OF ASTHMATIC ATTACKS

It is necessary, in order to understand what might be happening in asthma, to distinguish factors which *provoke* or *trigger* an individual episode of bronchoconstriction, from those which induce the '*asthmatic state*' in which airway hyper-responsiveness seems to be of paramount and central importance.

Non-specific triggers of bronchospasm, e.g. exercise, cold air hyperventilation, and fog can be expected to produce similar responses in all asthmatic subjects with similar levels of bronchial responsiveness[2]. The level of the stimulus, and the level of airway responsiveness are the only determinants of the severity of the bronchoconstrictor response. The mechanisms by which such triggers may operate will be dealt with later in the chapter.

In contrast to these non-specific stimuli, certain environmental agents provoke responses in only a proportion of those exposed, with no direct relation to the degree of non-specific airway responsiveness, although the latter may be an important determinant of the severity of the response. A specific 'sensitivity' to the agent seems to be involved. Classic immunological mechanisms or 'allergy' are probably responsible in most cases in which the agent is of organic origin, but this explanation probably does not apply to many of the reactive chemicals which cause 'occupational asthma', e.g. isocyanates, epoxyresins, formaldehyde, etc.

For both allergens and reactive chemicals, exposure of sensitized individuals leads to three separate, though almost certainly interrelated, events (Fig. 3.8):

(1) The *immediate asthmatic reaction* (IAR). Narrowing of the airways occurs with or shortly after exposure, reaching a maximum within 30 min and resolving spontaneously over the next 1–2 h. Airway smooth muscle contraction is largely responsible for the change in airway calibre.

(2) The *late asthmatic reaction* (LAR). Narrowing of the airways begins between one and 10 hours following exposure and reaches a maximum over several hours. It lasts for a variable number of hours, or even days in exceptional circumstances. Some of this airflow limitation is also due to muscle spasm, but oedema of the airway wall and mucus plugging is also thought to play an important, though ill-defined, part.

(3) *An increase in airway responsiveness.* A change occurs, as discussed above, *presumably* at the level of the smooth muscle fibre, which causes the airways to constrict at a level of stimulus (non-specific or pharmacological) to which they were previously unresponsive, either completely or relatively. This development of, or increase in, airway hyper-responsiveness is thought to be particularly associated with the LAR[13], although we do not know whether it is the LAR itself which causes responsiveness to change, or whether both are independent results of a more fundamental process. The recent demonstration that the change in responsiveness may occur before the LAR is suggestive of the latter[16].

Any model of the airway events underlying the responses to either allergen challenge or exposure to an industrial sensitizer

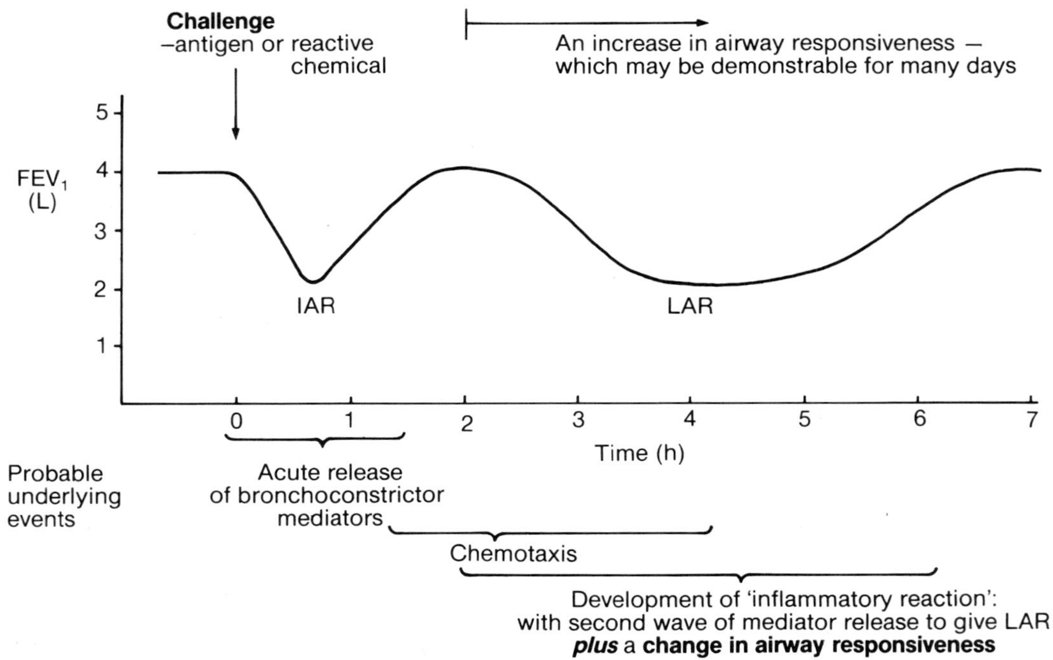

Figure 3.8 Time course of typical IAR and LAR after antigen or industrial 'sensitizer'

has to account for the whole sequence of responses. It also has to account for the fact that characteristically only a minority of exposed individuals develop any changes, and that some symptomatic individuals demonstrate only the IAR, others only the LAR and others both (i.e. a dual reaction). In addition, asthmatic reactions may develop in an individual only after months or years of repeated exposures.

For many environmental or occupational agents of organic origin that cause asthmatic reactions, the classical type I, IgE-mediated immune mechanism is central to the aetiology of the IAR. IgE is a specialized immunoglobulin class whose only physiological role is to bind, via its Fc fragment, to receptors on basophils, tissue mast cells and, it is now realized, macrophages and possibly also platelets. In this way these cells, once fixed by specific IgE molecules in sufficient numbers, become sensitized to subsequent antigen challenge. The reaction with a specific antigen involves cross-linking between adjacent IgE molecules, activation of the Fc receptor and configurational changes within the cell membrane which open cell membrane calcium channels. The resulting calcium influx causes cell activation and fusion of intracellular cytoplasmic granules with the cell membrane with release of a variety of preformed (stored) mediators, of which histamine is the archetype. This process is accompanied by the *de novo* generation of 'secondary' mediators, within the plasma membrane, consisting of PAF, and the families of prostaglandins, leukotrienes and related chemicals. Among the preformed and newly formed mediators there are not only potent smooth muscle contractile agents sufficient to cause the IAR, but also vasodilators, chemotaxins for neutrophils, eosinophils and platelets, activators of vagal reflexes and activators of axon reflexes with subsequent release of neuropeptides; in short, the panoply of agents necessary for the development of a full-blown inflammatory reaction (Fig. 3.9).

It is this inflammatory reaction, developing over the next few hours, with the generation of another wave of contractile chemicals that is almost certainly responsible for the LAR,

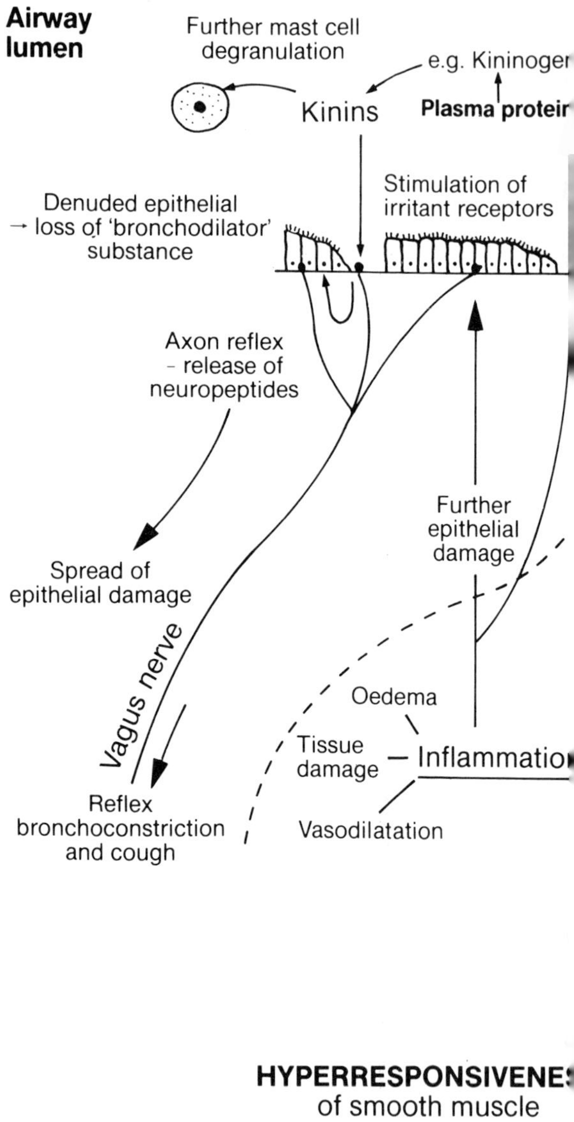

Airway lumen
Further mast cell degranulation
e.g. Kininogen
Kinins
Plasma protein
Stimulation of irritant receptors
Denuded epithelial → loss of 'bronchodilator' substance
Axon reflex - release of neuropeptides
Spread of epithelial damage
Further epithelial damage
Vagus nerve
Oedema
Tissue damage
Inflammation
Vasodilatation
Reflex bronchoconstriction and cough
HYPERRESPONSIVENESS of smooth muscle

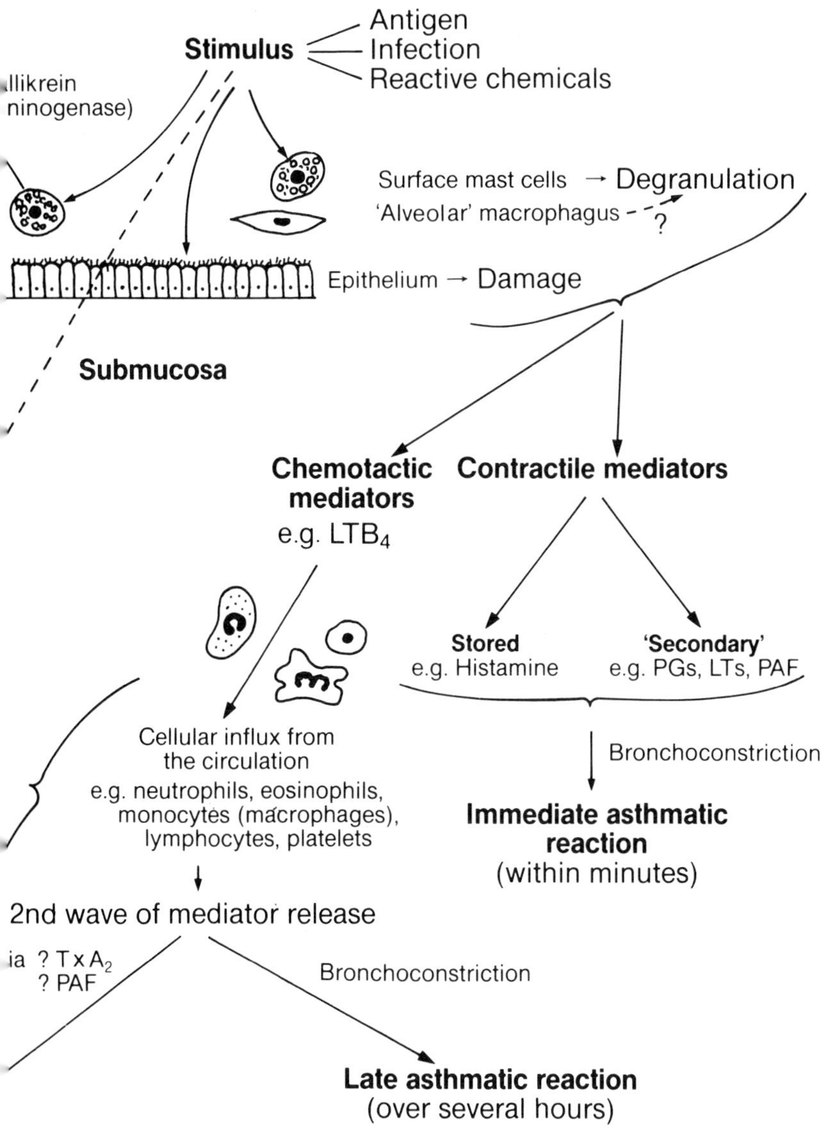

Figure 3.9 An 'inflammatory model' for the induction of airway hyper-responsiveness in humans

and, as discussed in detail above, for the induction of hyper-responsiveness.

The exact events which operate in the initiation of the asthmatic reaction to non-allergic agents are still unclear. It is probable, however, that the sequence of events and the end result is very much the same. Thus the 'insult' to the airway mucosa causes damage to a variety of cells, including probably mast cells, macrophages and epithelial cells with release of bronchoconstrictor mediators and chemotaxins, etc. in varying amounts. It is the balance of these mediators, between those causing *immediate bronchospasm* and those generating the later *inflammatory* reaction, that decides whether the patient will experience an IAR, a LAR (plus change in responsiveness) or a dual reaction.

Once these changes have occurred, with an increase in the responsiveness of the airways, the individual is then 'primed' for further exposures because subsequent reactions and release of mediators are increasingly likely to produce worsening clinical effects. The vulnerability of the airways may depend as well upon the presence of other intercurrent damaging and inflammatory events such as infection, noxious fumes, or coincidental immunological responses to other environmental agents. Thus, once initiated these events are likely to enter a vicious circle of pathological and clinical deterioration (Fig. 3.9).

REFERENCES

1. Hargreave, F. E., Juniper, E. F., Ryan, G., Dolovich, M., Cartier, A., Frith, P. A. and Newhouse, M. T. (1980). Clinical significance of non-specific airway hyper-reactivity. In: Hargreave, F. E. (ed) *Airway Reactivity. Mechanisms and clinical relevance.* pp. 216–22. (McMaster University)
2. Boushey, H. A., Holtzman, M. J., Sheller, J. R. and Nadel, J. A. (1980). Bronchial hyper-reactivity. *Am. Rev. Respir. Dis.,* **121,** 389–413
3. Orehek, J., Gayrard, P., Smith, A. P., Grimaud, C. and Charpin, J. (1977). Airway response to carbachol in normal and asthmatic subjects. *Am. Rev. Resp. Dis.,* **115,** 937–43
4. Cockcroft, D. W., Killian, D. N., Mellon, J. J. A. and Hargreave, F. E. (1977). Bronchial reactivity to inhaled histamine: a method and clinical survey. *Clin. Allergy,* **7,** 235–43

5. Chai, H., Farr, R. S., Froelich, L. A., Mathison, D. A., McLean, J. A., Rosenthal, R. R., Sheffer, A. L., Spector, S. L. and Townley, R. G. (1975). Standardisation of bronchial inhalation challenge procedures. *J. Allergy Clin. Immunol.*, **56,** 331–7
6. Ryan, G., Dolovich, M. B., Roberts, R. S., Frith, P. A., Juniper, E. F., Hargreave, F. E. and Newhouse, M. T. (1981). Standardisation of inhalation provocation tests: two techniques of aerosol generation and inhalation compared. *Am. Rev. Resp. Dis.*, **123,** 195–9
7. Brittan, J., Mortagy, A. and Tattersfield, A. (1986). Histamine challenge tests: comparison of three methods. *Thorax*, **41,** 128–32
8. Juniper, E. F., Frith, P. A. and Hargreave, F. E. (1981). Airway responsiveness to histamine and methacholine: relationship to minimum treatment to control symptoms of asthma. *Thorax*, **36,** 575–9
9. Chatham, M., Bleecker, E. R., Smith, P. L., Rosenthal, R. R., Mason, P. and Norman, P. S. A comparison of histamine, methacholine, and exercise airway reactivity in normal and asthmatic subjects. *Am. Rev. Resp. Dis.*, **126,** 235–40
10. Burney, P. G. J., Britton, J. R., Chinn, S., Tattersfield, A. E., Papacosta, A. O., Kelson, M. C., Anderson, F. and Corfield, D. R. (1987). Descriptive epidemiology of bronchial reactivity in an adult population: results from a community study. *Thorax*, **42,** 38–44
11. Chung, K. F. (1986). Role of inflammation in the hyper-reactivity of the airways in asthma. *Thorax*, **41,** 657–62
12. Empey, D. W., Laitinen, L. A., Jacobs, L., Gold, W. H. and Nadel, J. A. (1976). Mechanisms of bronchial hyper-reactitivy in normal subjects after upper respiratory tract infections. *Am. Rev. Resp. Dis.*, **113,** 131–9
13. Cockcroft, D. W., Ruffin, R. E., Dolovich, J. and Hargreave, F. E. (1977). Allergen-induced increase in non-allergic bronchial reactivity. *Clin. Allergy*, **7,** 503–13
14. Golden, J. A., Nadel, J. A., Boushey, H. A. (1978). Bronchial hyper-irritability in health subjects after exposure to ozone. *Am. Rev. Resp. Dis.*, **118,** 287–94
15. Mink, J. T., Gerrard, J. W., Cockcroft, D. W., Cotton, D. J. and Dosman, J. A. (1980). Increased bronchial reactivity to inhaled histamine in non-smoking grain workers with normal lung function. *Chest*, **77,** 28–31
16. Durham, S. R., Graneek, B. J., Hawkins, R. and Newman-Taylor, A. J. The temporal relationship between increases in airway responsiveness to histamine and late asthmatic responses induced by occupational gents. *J. Allergy Clin. Immunol.* (in Press)
17. Barnes, P. J. (1986). Neural control of human airways in health and disease. *Am. Rev. Resp. Dis.*, **134,** 1289–1314
18. Florey, H. Secretion of mucus in the inflammation of mucous membranes. (1982). In: Florey, H. (ed) *General pathology*. 3rd ed. pp. 1962–6. (London: Lloyd-Duke (Medical Books))
19. Dunnill, M. S. (1960). The pathology of asthma with special reference to changes in the bronchial mucosa. *J. Clin. Pathol.*, **13,** 27–33

20. Laitinen, L. A., Heino, M., Laitinen, A., Kava, T. and Haahtela, T. (1985). Damage of the airway epithelium and bronchial reactivity in patients with asthma. *Am. Rev. Resp. Dis.*, **131,** 599–606
21. Godard, P. G., Chaintreuil, J., Damon, M., Coupe, M., Flandre, O., Castes de Paulet, A. and Michel, F. B. (1982). Functional assessment of alveolar macrophages: comparison of cells from asthmatics and normal subjects. *J. Allergy Clin. Immunol.*, **70,** 88–93
22. Holtzman, M. J., Fabbri, L. M., Skoogh, B. E., O'Byrne, P. M., Walters, E. H., Aizawa, H. and Nadel, J. A. (1983). Time course of airway hyper-responsiveness induced by ozone in dogs. *J. Appl. Physiol.*, **54,** 134–9
23. Golden, J. A., Nadel, J. A. and Boushey, H. (1978). Bronchial hyper-irritability in healthy subjects after exposure to ozone. *Am. Rev. Resp. Dis.*, **118,** 287–94
24. Holtzman, M. J., Fabbri, L. M., O'Byrne, P. M., Gold, D. B., Aizawa, H., Walters, E. H., Alpert, S. E. and Nadel, J. A. (1983). Importance of airway inflammation for hyper-responsiveness induced by ozone. *Am. Rev. Resp. Dis.*, **127,** 686–90
25. Fabbri, L. M., Aizawa, H. A., Alpert, S. E., Walters, E. H., O'Byrne, P. M., Nadel, J. A. and Holtzman, M. J. (1984). Airway hyper-responsiveness and changes of cell count in bronchoalveolar lavage after ozone in dogs. *Am. Rev. Resp. Dis.*, **129,** 288–91
26. Holtzman, M. J., Aizawa, H., Nadel, J. A. and Goetzl, E. J. (1983). Selective generation of leukotriene B4 by tracheal epithelial cells from dogs. *Biochem. Biophys. Res. Commun.*, **114,** 1071–6
27. O'Byrne, P. M., Walters, E. H., Gold, D. B., Aizawa, H. A., Fabbri, L. M., Alpert, S. E., Nadel, J. A. and Holtzman, M. J. (1984). Neutrophil depletion inhibits airway hyper-responsiveness induced by ozone exposure. *Am. Rev. Resp. Dis.*, **130,** 214–9
28. O'Byrne, P. M., Walters, E. H., Fabbri, L. M., Holtzman, M. J and Nadel, J. A. (1984). Indomethacin inhibits the airway hyper-responsiveness but not the neutrophil influx induced by ozone in dogs. *Am. Rev. Resp. Dis.*, **130,** 220–4
29. Aizawa, H., Chung, K. F., Leikauf, G. D., Ueki, I., Bethel, R. A., O'Byrne, P. M., Hirose, T. and Nadel, J. A. (1985). Significance of thromboxane generation in ozone-induced airway hyper-responsiveness in dogs. *J. Appl. Physiol.*, **59,** 1918–23
30. O'Byrne, P. M., Leikauf, G. D., Aizawa, H., Bethel, R. A., Ueki, I. F., Holtzman, M. J. and Nadel, J. A. (1985). Leukotriene B4 induces airway hyper-responsiveness in dogs. *J. Appl. Physiol.*, **59,** 1941–6
31. Chung, K. F., Becker, A. B., Lazarus, S. C., Fick, O. L., Nadel, J. A. and Gold, W. M. (1985). Antigen-induced airway hyper-responsiveness and pulmonary inflammation in allergic dogs. *J. Appl. Physiol.*, **58,** 1347–53
32. Murlas, C. G. and Roum, J. H. (1985). Sequence of pathologic changes in the airway mucosa of guinea pigs during ozone-induced bronchial hyper-reactivity. *Am. Rev. Resp. Dis.*, **131,** 314–20
33. Hulbert, W. C., Walker, D. C., Jackson, A. and Hogg, J. C. (1981). Airway permeability to horseradish peroxidase in guinea pigs: the repair

phase after injury by cigarette smoke. *Am. Rev. Resp. Dis.*, **123,** 320–6
34. Gordon, T., Sheppard, D., McDonald, D. M., Distefono, S. and Scypinski, L. (1985). Airway hyper-responsiveness and inflammation induced by toluene di-isocyanate in guinea pigs. *Am. Rev. Resp. Dis.*, **132,** 1106–12
35. De Monchy, J. G. R., Kauffman, H. F., Venge, P., Koeter, G. H., Jansen, H. M., Sluiter, H. J. and de Vries, K. (1985). Bronchoalveolar eosinophils during allergen-induced late asthmatic reactions. *Am. Rev. Resp. Dis*, **131,** 373–6
36. Durham, S. R. and Kay, A. B. (1985). Eosinophils, bronchial hyperreactivity and late-phase asthmatic reactions. *Clin. Allergy*, **15,** 411–8
37. Seltzer, J., Bigby, B. G., Stulbarg, M., Holtzman, M. J., Nadel, J. A., Ueki, I. F., Leikauf, G. D., Goetzl, E. J. and Boushey, H. A. (1986). Ozone induced change in bronchial reactivity to methacholine and airway inflammation in human subjects. *J. Appl. Physiol.*, **60,** 1321–6
38. Fabbri, L. M., Boschetto, P., Zocca, E. and Milani, G. F. (1987). Bronchoalveolar neutrophilia during TDI-induced late asthmatic reactions. *Am. Rev. Resp. Dis.* (In Press)
39. Flint, K. C., Leung, K. B. P., Hudspith, B. N., Brostoff, J., Pearce, F. L. and Johnson, N. M. (1985). Bronchoalveolar mast cells in extrinsic asthma: a mechanism for the initiation of antigen specific bronchoconstriction. *Br. Med. J.*, **291,** 923–6
40. Metzger, W. J., Hunninghake, G. W. and Richerson, H. B. (1985). Late asthmatic responses: inquiry into mechanisms and significance. *Clin. Rev. Allergy*, **3,** 145–65
41. Knauer, K. A., Lichtenstein, L. M., Adkinson, F. N. and Fish, J. E. (1981). Platelet activation during antigen-induced airway reactions in asthmatic subjects. *N. Engl. J. Med.*, **304,** 1404–7
42. Joseph, M., Auriault, C., Capron, A., Vorng, H. and Viens, P. (1983). A new function for platelets: IgE-dependent killing of schistosomes. *Nature*, **303,** 310–2
43. Walters, E. H., Parrish, R. W., Bevan, C. and Smith, A. P. (1981). Induction of bronchial hypersensitivity: evidence for a role for prostaglandins. *Thorax*, **36,** 571–4
44. Fuller, R. W., Dixon, C. M. S., Dollery, C. T. and Barnes, P. J. (1986). Prostaglandin D_2 potentiates airway responsiveness to histamine and methacholine. *Am. Rev. Resp. Dis.*, **133,** 252–4
45. Walters, E. H., Bevan, C, Parrish, R. W., Davies, B. H. and Smith, A. P. (1982). Time dependent effect of PGE_2 inhalation upon airway responses to bronchoconstrictor agents in normal subjects. *Thorax*, **37,** 438–42
46. Cuss, F. M., Dixon, C. M. and Barnes, P. J. (1986). Inhaled platelet activating factor in man: effects on pulmonary function and bronchial responsiveness. *Lancet*, **2,** 189–92
47. Chung, K. F., Aizawa, H., Leikauf, G. D., Heki, I. F., Evans, T. W. and Nadel, J. A. (1986) Airway hyper-responsiveness induced by platelet-activating factor: role of thromboxane generation. *J. Pharmacol. Exp. Ther.*, **236,** 580–4
48. Christiansen, S. C., Proud, D. and Chochrane, C. G. (1987). Detection

of tissue kallikrein in the bronchoalveolar lavage fluid of asthmatic subjects. *J. Clin. Invest.*, **79,** 188–97
49. Barnes, P. J. (1986). Asthma as an axon reflex. *Lancet*, **1,** 242–5
50. Walters, E. H. (1983). Prostaglandins and the control of airway responses to histamine in normal and asthmatic subjects. *Thorax*, **38,** 188–94
51. Walters, E. H. (1983). Effect of inhibition of prostaglandin synthesis on induced bronchial hyper-responsiveness. *Thorax*, **38,** 195–9
52. Fujimura, M., Sasaki, F., Nakatsumi, Y., Takahashi, Y., Hifumi, S, Taga, K., Mifune, J. I., Tonaka, T. and Matsuda, T. (1986). Effects of a thromboxane synthetase inhibitor (OKY046) and a lipoxygenase inhibitor (AA-861) on bronchial responsiveness to acetylcholine in asthmatic subjects. *Thorax*, **41,** 955–9
53. Copas, J. L., Borgeat, P. and Gardiner, P. J. (1982). The actions of 5-, 12- and 15-HETE on tracheobronchial smooth muscle. *Prostaglandin Leuk. Med.*, **8,** 105–14
54. Vinenc, K. S., Black, J. L., Yan, K., Armour, C. L., Donnelly, P. D. and Woolcock, A. J. (1983). Comparison of *in vivo* and *in vitro* responses to histamine in human airways. *Am. Rev. Resp. Dis.*, **128,** 875–9
55. Roberts, J. A., Raeburn, D., Rudger, I. W. and Thomson, N. C. (1984). Comparison of *in vivo* airway responsiveness and *in vitro* smooth muscle sensitivity to methacholine in man. *Thorax*, **39,** 837–43
56. Walters, E. H., O'Byrne, P. M., Graf, P. D., Fabbri, L. M. and Nadel, J. A. (1986). The responsiveness of airway smooth muscle *in vitro* from dogs with airway hyper-responsiveness *in vivo*. *Clin. Sci.*, **71,** 605–11
57. Walters, E. H., O'Byrne, P. M., Fabbri, L. M., Graf, P. D., Holtzman, M. J. and Nadel, J. A. (1984). Control of neurotransmission by prostaglandins in canine trachealis smooth muscle. *J. Appl. Physiol.*, **57,** 129–34
58. Chung, K. F., Evans, T. W., Graf, P. D. and Nadel, J. A. (1985). Modulation of cholinergic neurotransmission in canine airways by thromboxane-mimetic U46619. *Eur. J. Pharmacol.*, **117,** 373–5
59. Boulet, L. P., Latimer, K. M., Roberts, R. S., Juniper, E. F., Cockcroft, D. W., Thomson, N. C., Daniel, E. E. and Hargreave, F. E. (1984). The effect of atropine on allergen-induced increases in bronchial responsiveness to histamine. *Am. Rev. Resp. Dis.*, **130,** 318–22
60. Barnes, P. J., Cuss, F. M. C. and Palmer, J. B. D. (1985). The effect of airway epithelium on smooth muscle contractility in bovine trachea. *Br. J. Pharmacol.*, **86,** 685–91

4

THE TREATMENT OF ASTHMA

INTRODUCTION

The options available for the treatment of asthma have increased over the last ten to twenty years. New groups of agents have been introduced, and the choice within groups such as the beta agonists has increased. For many of these drugs there has been a change in the method of administration. Within the beta agonists and the corticosteroids there has been a move towards inhaled therapy with the development of more devices for inhalation. This has the advantage of allowing the use of much smaller doses of the active agent and reducing undesirable side-effects. Within other groups of drugs, such as the theophyllines, improvement in the release characteristics of the oral formulation has allowed better control of oral therapy.

Associated with this increased choice of pharmacological agents has come a greater interest in non-pharmacological methods of control. Techniques such as acupuncture, hypnotherapy and relaxation therapies have begun to be assessed in scientifically valid trials which will enable them to be genuinely evaluated.

Attention has also begun to turn to an understanding of the

importance of patient education and compliance with therapy. As with many other treatments of chronic diseases, compliance with asthmatic therapy is often poor. It is all very well to have an effective prophylactic therapy but it is of little use unless the patient takes it appropriately. Education to overcome this is likely to be increasingly important if there is to be a shift towards prophylactic controlling therapy for asthma, rather than just therapy which responds in acute exacerbations. The first part of this chapter will cover the available options for treatment, and the second half will concentrate on the management of particular forms of asthma.

AVAILABLE TREATMENTS FOR ASTHMA

Bronchodilators

Beta agonists

1. Mechanism of action. Sympathomimetic agents have been used in the treatment of asthma for over eighty years, ever since adrenaline was first shown to be active. Long before this, ephedrine had been used in Far Eastern medicine. The recognition of different sorts of adrenergic receptors, the α_1, α_2, β_1 and β_2 receptors, has been followed by the development of drugs specifically acting on different receptors. Beta$_1$-receptors are found mainly on cardiac muscle and smooth muscle of the gut. Beta$_2$-receptors are located on airway smooth muscle, skeletal muscle, uterine muscle and the smooth muscle in the walls of blood vessels. The bronchial smooth muscle has little if any direct sympathetic innervation but it has plentiful β-receptors[1]. Stimulation of the β-receptor stimulates the enzyme adenyl cyclase, which increases the formation of cyclic AMP (3, 5-cyclic adenosine monophosphate) from ATP (adenosine triphosphate). The tone in the bronchial smooth muscle is regulated by the balance between cyclic AMP and cyclic GMP, which is produced by stimulation of the parasympathetic system. Cyclic AMP leads to the activation of protein kinases which inhibit the contractile mechanism of myosin and reduce intracellular calcium. There has recently been increasing interest in non-adrenergic and non-cholinergic nerves in the airway smooth muscle, but specific pharmacological agents to work on these systems are not yet available. The generation of cyclic AMP also decreases mediator release from mast cells and decreases oedema from the mucosa.

2. *Specificity.* The specific β_2-receptor agonist salbutamol was introduced in 1969, and a number of other selective β-stimulants have appeared since then (Table 4.1). With the advent of these selective drugs, there is little reason to continue using the earlier non-selective agents in current therapy. The commonest selective agents now in use are salbutamol, terbutaline, fenoterol and rimiterol. When they are given by inhalation, these drugs have a rapid onset of action, producing most of their peak effect within 15 minutes of administration. Rimiterol may have a slightly faster onset but also has a relatively short half-life and is beginning to lose its effect soon after the first hour. The other drugs have similar time courses of action, beginning to lose their effect between four to six hours. The many types of inhalation devices now available, including metered dose inhalers, dry powder inhalers, spacer devices and nebulizers mean that nearly every patient is able to use β-receptor agents by the inhaled route[1]. This leaves little

Table 4.1 Selective β-stimulants for inhalation

Drug	*Dose per actuation* (μg)
Salbutamol	100 (+200 and 400 rotacaps)
Terbutaline	250
Fenoterol	180
Pirbuterol	200
Reproterol	500
Rimiterol	200 (breath actuated unit available)

place for oral β-stimulant drugs, since these have the same sort of length of action as inhaled therapy but a slower onset and a much higher incidence of side effects[2].

Practical point

- The various devices available for inhalation mean that almost all patients can use inhaled drugs

3. Oral administration. Occasional patients may benefit from the use of slow release oral preparations for nocturnal symptoms, and there may also be a place for oral therapy in the treatment of young children who find inhalers difficult to handle. The use of oral drugs has declined over the last ten years with the advent of the inhalation devices. The dose administered is ten to twenty times the amount delivered by a metered dose inhaler.

4. Side effects. The side-effects most often encountered with inhaled therapy are fine tremor, feelings of anxiety and occasional tachycardia. These side-effects are not troublesome in the majority of patients. With oral therapy, side-effects are more likely to be a problem, and other muscle problems, such as cramp, may also occur. Administration of β-receptor agonists can lead to a reduction in serum potassium, although this has even been used as a treatment of hyperkalaemic periodic paralysis, but it is rarely a problem except with parenteral therapy. Angina and cardiac arrhythmias can be precipitated by the larger doses delivered by nebulizers[3], and in those known to have ischaemic heart disease the nebulizer dose should be kept low, e.g. 2.5 mg salbutamol.

The increase in asthma deaths which occurred in the 1960s was associated by some workers with the introduction of the non-specific β-agonist aerosols, particularly isoprenaline. However, subsequent analysis of this data has suggested that this was probably not the case. Nevertheless, there is a danger with any effective bronchodilator that because this is usually extremely effective, patients may continue to use the treatment rather than seek further appropriate help during acute severe exacerbations of asthma. This danger has been proposed as a potential problem with the use of home nebulizers for asthma, and certainly careful patient selection and education is essential for such use[4].

5. *Nebulizers.* A number of the β-agonists are available as nebulizer solutions. Nebulizers can deliver large doses directly to the lungs. However, as with metered dose inhalers, only a small proportion of the drug in the nebulizer chamber actually reaches the intrapulmonary airways. With metered dose inhalers most of the loss occurs by impaction in the oropharynx, while with nebulizers most of the loss is within the nebulizer tubing and from nebulization during expiration. Approximately 12% of the drug in the nebulizer chamber goes into the lungs. Nebulizers have a number of uses and are not used only to give bronchodilators (Table 4.2).

Table 4.2 Uses of nebulizers

1. To deliver drugs in those unable to use other inhalation devices
2. To deliver large doses of bronchodilator regularly
3. To treat acute asthma.

Children who find it difficult to use metered dose inhalers and dry powder systems can be given regular therapy with sodium cromoglycate, corticosteroids and bronchodilators. Sometimes, cheaper spacer devices can provide an alternative.

The dose response curves of most normal and asthmatic subjects show maximum responses to quite low doses of β-agonists, often at or below 100 μg salbutamol or its equivalent. However, some patients do show increased responses with higher doses, sometimes up to around 5 mg salbutamol. In some such patients nebulizers provide the most convenient way of delivering these doses. This form of chronic nebulizer use can be evaluated by symptom diaries and peak flow monitoring.

In acute attacks of asthma nebulizers are an important, safe part of therapy for use by general practitioners, ambulance crew and hospitals, but their use at home by asthmatics for acute exacerbations is more debatable. It is in this situation that the greatest dangers exist and raise, as with isoprenaline inhalers, the possibility that patients may stay at home using this therapy which is usually effective, rather than seeking further essential emergency care.

6. *Tachyphylaxis.* The question of loss of effect of bronchodilator action with continued use, or tachyphylaxis, has been widely investigated. There is some conflicting data available, but the overall conclusion of these studies is that even if tachyphylaxis does occur with continuing therapy, its effects are only minor and are quickly removed by a brief period off the drug or by corticosteroid therapy[5]. It is interesting that the airways seem to be relatively protected from this tachyphylaxis since reduction in activity is comparatively easy to demonstrate in tremor and peripheral lymphocyte β-receptors. There is no reason to think there are any particular differences between the various selective β-agonists in their incidence of side-effects or in tachyphylaxis. However, there are many anecdotes suggesting that occasional patients do seem to find trouble with tremor on one agent which does not occur on switching to an alternative drug. Such side-effects may also disappear with continued therapy.

7. *Parenteral use.* Some of these β-receptor agonists are also available for parenteral therapy. Terbutaline and salbutamol are most often used in this way. They can be used subcutaneously, intramuscularly or intravenously in acute exacerbations of asthma. In most cases there seems no advantage to be gained from giving the drug parenterally rather than by nebulization. However, there are situations when it may be easier to administer subcutaneous or intramuscular injections. Occasional asthmatic patients have such acute severe attacks that they need to be taught to carry this therapy with them and to administer such injections for themselves. There has also been interest in the administration of β-agonists by con-

tinuous subcutaneous infusion. This method provides effective treatment but blood levels seem to indicate that the results are related to the delivery of high doses of the drugs.

Anticholinergic agents

Anticholinergic drugs have long been known to be effective in relieving bronchoconstriction. Deadly nightshade extracts (*Atropa belladonna*) and thornapple (*Datnea stramonium*) have formed traditional remedies. Stramonium made up the active ingredient of asthma cigarettes. They act by blocking vagal bronchoconstricting activity and the effects of general vagal blockade limit their use to the inhaled route. The main compound available for many years was atropine, in the form of sulphate or methonitrate. More recently, most anticholinergic treatment has been with ipratropium bromide, which was introduced in the mid-1970s. These agents act by competitive antagonism of acetylcholine, reducing the activity of guanyl cyclase and decreasing the formation of cyclic GMP (guanosine 5-monophosphate). One of the worries of anticholinergic therapy has been that it might dry airway secretions, reduce mucociliary clearance and contribute to mucus plugging. Ipratropium bromide has been found not to have these effects, and has a degree of selectivity for the bronchi rather than the heart and salivary glands[5]. It is available for inhaled therapy only, in the form of metered dose inhaler and nebulized solution. In the initial management of acute asthma, ipratropium bromide has been found to be as effective as salbutamol[6]. In studies outside acute exacerbations, and in exercise-induced asthma, ipratropium bromide often turns out to be less successful than β-stimulants in the management of asthma. However, in older patients with more persistent chronic airflow obstruction, ipratropium bromide may be more effective and may also produce an additional effect on top of the bronchodilating abilities of maximal doses of β-agonists[7]. In children below eighteen months β-agonists may fail to produce bronchodilatation, while nebulization of ipratropium bromide may be effective.

Inhaled ipratropium bromide has a slower onset of action than β-agonists. It takes 30 to 60 minutes to reach its maximal effect, but the action is more prolonged and lasts for six to eight hours. Apart from a bitter taste on inhalation, the only occasional problem with ipratropium bromide is paradoxical bronchoconstriction.

Occasional patients have been noticed to develop airway narrowing after administration of ipratropium bromide from a metered dose inhaler. The reason for this is uncertain but it has been suggested that it may be related to the bromide radical. When used as nebulized therapy, adverse reactions to ipratropium bromide seem to have been slightly more frequent. Initial results suggest that these effects were more frequent when a hypotonic preparation of the nebulizer solution was available, and when dilution was made with distilled water rather than normal saline. Problems were diminished by changing the formulation to an isotonic preparation and diluting in normal saline[8]. However, it has been suggested that such reactions may still occasionally occur in patients with markedly increased airway reactivity even with isotonic ipratropium bromide, and that this may be related to preservatives in the nebulizer solution. These events are rare, but do mean that a first inhalation of ipratropium bromide should be given under supervision. Such reactions are very occasionally seen with the administration of β-receptor agonists, particularly in very young children. It may be that, in general, these events are much less likely to be seen with β-agonists because of the faster onset of action of the bronchodilatation covering any possible adverse reactions.

Methylxanthines

The methylxanthines are plant alkaloids and consist of a group of three naturally occurring substances, theophylline, theobromine and caffeine. Although theobromine and caffeine can be found to have bronchodilatory properties, by far the most important agent in this group is theophylline. Combination of theophylline with ethylenediamine produces the soluble form aminophylline. Diprophylline is a substituted theophylline and suprophylline is a non-methylated xanthine. The mechanism of action of methylxanthines in producing bronchodilatation is disputed.

Theophylline can be administered orally, rectally or parenterally[9]. A large number of sustained-release preparations for oral therapy is now available. These have various release characteristics. They are designed to try to produce steady blood levels and have been developed in response to the recognition of the difficulties of theophylline therapy. The therapeutic range of theophylline is usually described as being within 8 to 20 mg/l. While effectiveness may increase through this range and even above these levels, the incidence of side-effects rises. The commonest side-effect is gastrointestinal irritation with nausea and vomiting. In some subjects these effects occur within this therapeutic range, so that there is little safety margin between the therapeutic and toxic effects of theophylline. The situation is further complicated by marked individual differences in absorption and metabolism of theophylline, and interaction with various other drugs (Table 4.3).

These problems make individual prediction of levels from the doses given difficult. A number of studies have found that when levels are checked from patients on theophylline therapy, either in routine outpatient follow-up or presenting with acute asthma, many of them have levels below the therapeutic range[10]. A minority are found to have toxic levels and once more this is unpredictable and provides problems in giving intravenous aminophylline to those already on oral therapy.

These difficulties mean that most UK physicians do not see theophyllines as first-line bronchodilator therapy but much prefer to use safer inhaled treatment. However, there is no doubt that methylxanthines are effective and, in certain circumstances, their use is desirable. They have been shown to be effective for nocturnal asthma[11], and may be used for children where inhaled therapy is more difficult to administer

Table 4.3 Drugs interacting with theophylline

Increased clearance (dose may need to be increased)
Enzyme-inducers
phenobarbitone
phenytoin
rifampicin
ethanol
carbamazepine
Tobacco
Marihuana
Decreased clearance (dose may need to be reduced)
Enzyme-inhibitors
cimetidine
oral contraceptive
erythromycin
β-blockers
Caffeine
Influenza vaccine

and may even be less effective. In order to get the dosing of theophylline right, it is advisable to check on the blood level of theophylline being achieved. Levels should be taken daily while on continuous intravenous therapy for acute asthma. During chronic oral treatment levels can be measured about one week after starting a given dose. Subsequently, with no significant change in renal, hepatic or cardiac function and no drug interactions, a repeat level once or twice a year is adequate. The drugs shown in Table 4.3 interact with theophylline.

For parenteral use theophylline is given as the-ethylenediamine salt, aminophylline. This can be given as a bolus dose, but only as a slow intravenous infusion over 15 to 30 minutes. This can be followed up with a continuous intravenous infusion. The dosage should be adjusted according to the size of the patient, the interacting factors shown in Table

4.3, the presence of previous theophylline treatment, and by monitoring theophylline levels.

Administration of theophylline by the rectal route results in a rapid increase in blood levels since the portal venous system is bypassed. However, the absorption is unpredictable and proctitis is a common complication.

Prophylactic Therapy

The bronchodilator drugs described above can all be used as prophylactic therapy, and in this way will prevent the onset of many attacks of asthma. They have often been used as regular long-term therapy in this way. Drugs such as β-stimulants are very effective in preventing the onset of asthma in response to specific stimuli in the laboratory. For instance, they are the best drug available for the prevention of exercise-induced asthma[12]. A number of other drugs are now available which, while they do not have a bronchodilator action in reversing acute bronchoconstriction, do have a longer-term suppressive action in controlling asthma by preventing the onset of problems. The recognition that even patients whose asthma is well controlled appear to have continuing pathological damage in the airways has led to the suggestion that these drugs, which may have an anti-inflammatory effect, are particularly important in reducing the long-term damage of asthma. This has been related to their effect in reducing the non-specific bronchial reactivity of the airways to substances such as methacholine and histamine.

This property of reducing bronchial reactivity which is seen with sodium cromoglycate and inhaled steroids is not shared by long-term use of bronchodilators. Recognition has increased that poorly controlled asthma can lead to permanent lung damage and the development of irreversible airflow obstruction. This important concept of treatment, which may if true lead to the prevention of the consequences of many years of uncontrolled asthma, is potentially of great consequence.

However, it remains to be satisfactorily proven in valid long-term studies. The suggestion has even been made that the use of bronchodilators alone might increase this pathological damage by allowing continued exposure to irritants and allergens without affecting the inflammatory changes.

Sodium Cromoglycate

Sodium cromoglycate was introduced in 1967, and was thought to act by preventing the release of mediators from mast cells by stopping the reaction provoked by the combination of allergen with specific IgE at the cell surface. This involves blockade of the influx of calcium and cytoplasmic phosphodiesterase inhibition. Once again, doubt has been raised as to the precise mechanism of sodium cromoglycate, but it remains an effective drug in many patients. It appears to be particularly effective in children with a substantial allergic component in their asthma. In the laboratory, sodium cromoglycate also blocks bronchoconstriction induced by non-allergic stimuli such as exercise, irritant gases and hyperventilation.

In general, it needs to be taken as continuous therapy. It has no effect in the treatment of acute attacks of asthma. Although it can be used as a prophylactic to avoid the onset of exercise-induced asthma, its action in this regard is not as reliable as that of β-agonists[12]. Sodium cromoglycate is effective in some adults in producing control of the asthma, even if there are no apparent allergic triggers. Usually it needs to be used for one to two months to develop its effects. The introduction of inhaled corticosteroids and the reassurance about the general lack of side-effects of their use has diminished the role of sodium cromoglycate, which is often rather less effective as suppressive therapy. Nevertheless, there remains a number of children who can be very adequately controlled with regular sodium cromoglycate therapy. There is little evidence that sodium cromoglycate adds anything to control once the decision has been taken to start on inhaled corticosteroids.

The original use of sodium cromoglycate was as a dry powder administered by way of a spinhaler. It has been available as a dry powder alone or as Intal compound in combination with a small amount of isoprenaline. The isoprenaline was introduced to deal with the immediate bronchoconstriction which can occur in some asthmatics with the inhalation of dry powder. Problems with the compound preparation come from the misunderstanding of its use among patients. Because the isoprenaline has an acute bronchodilating effect, it may become used for this action rather than in a regular fashion for its suppressive sodium cromoglycate effect. Newer preparations of sodium cromoglycate have come as metered dose inhalers in 1 mg and 5 mg strengths. The usual dose of sodium cromoglycate in adults is one spincap, or 5–10 mg, by metered dose inhaler four times a day. Apart from the occasional irritation and bronchoconstriction there are virtually no side-effects from the use of sodium cromoglycate.

Nedocromil Sodium

Since the introduction of sodium cromoglycate in the 1960s, many attempts have been made to develop similar drugs, but few have come to fruition. Nedocromil sodium was released in 1986. It appears to have a similar action to sodium cromoglycate, with the addition of an anti-inflammatory effect. This wider basis of action means that nedocromil sodium may work in a broader range of patients. Once again it appears to be less effective than moderate doses of inhaled corticosteroids, but it provides a useful adjunct to the range of options available in this approach to the management of asthma. It is likely that a number of other similar drugs will become available in the next few years. Those under development include antagonists of leukotrienes, membrane derived mediators from mast cells.

Antihistamines

Antihistamines, which might be expected to be effective in asthma, have been disappointing, having little if any effect, in contrast to their benefit in allergic rhinitis. This may well be related to the number of mediators involved in the asthmatic process so that antagonism of one single element is ineffective.

Ketotifen

Ketotifen is an oral drug which is related to antihistamines but was introduced not because of its H_1 blocking activity, but because *in vitro* it appeared to have actions similar to sodium cromoglycate. As with many drugs in this group, it has been difficult to prove its effectiveness because of the chronicity of the treatment required, and the intrinsic variability of asthma. Overall, it has not proved particularly effective and has a significant incidence of sedation as a side-effect.

Calcium antagonists

Interest in the role of calcium in smooth muscle activity has increased with the realization of its fundamental role in contraction processes. The calcium antagonist drugs verapamil and nifedipine, which have been effective in reducing vascular smooth muscle, have been investigated but have not been shown to have any useful effect in the management of asthma. They do not have any bronchodilator action, although they do appear to have a minor effect on partially preventing exercise-induced asthma and reaction to non-specific airway challenge, with agents such as histamine. This in itself may not be a beneficial effect in the treatment of asthma, but it does mean that these drugs provide a safe alternative to β-blockers in the management of hypertension and angina. Beta-blockers should not be used in asthmatic patients. The so-called selective agents are not nearly selective enough to be safe and even the use of β-blocker eye drops has been associated with fatal reactions in asthmatics.

Corticosteroids

Corticosteroids are hydrocortisone analogues which bind selectively to glucocorticoid receptors. They hold an important place in the management of asthma. Despite this, intense investigation has failed to discover with certainty their mode of action. Messenger RNA is produced in response to stimulation of specific DNA chromatin. This process takes some hours and may explain the slow onset of the corticosteroid effect in acute asthma. There is blockade of the synthesis and release of various mediators and airway inflammation is reduced. The synthesis and release of an inhibitory protein known as lipomodulin are increased. The lipomodulin reduces the generation of mediators from arachidonic acid. There is an additional effect on calcium transport. The relative importance of these various mechanisms is uncertain.

Oral corticosteroids. Oral corticosteroids have been shown to be effective in the control of deteriorating asthma, treatment of acute attacks of asthma, and the long-term control of chronic asthma. However, the well-known side-effects from long-term treatment with corticosteroids mean that they must be handled with circumspection, and the emergence of inhaled corticosteroids has enabled many patients to avoid the problems of long-term chronic therapy with oral drugs. In general, it is undesirable for asthmatics to be on treatment with continuous oral corticosteroids. Earlier reports that asthmatics on corticosteroids might be protected from osteoporosis have proved false. They are prone to exactly the same effects as patients with other diseases on this treatment[13]. Nevertheless, in occasional patients long-term use is essential.

A very different approach should be maintained to the use of short courses of corticosteroids for deteriorating asthma and acute exacerbations. This provides a life saving treatment. The majority of studies into asthma deaths has shown that nearly all deaths are associated with undertreatment rather than overtreatment[14], and the principal worry in these studies has been the fact that most asthmatics who die fail to get onto treatment with steroids when their asthma is deteriorating premorbidly. The failure to start corticosteroid treatment comes from a combination of inadequate recognition of the potential severity of asthma on the part of patients, general practitioners and hospital doctors.

Asthmatics who have shown a tendency to have severe attacks can generally be taught to control their own steroid therapy, keeping a supply at home to start when the need arises. They are likely to become increasingly confident in their use of such courses if they have an objective measure of their asthma available to supplement their subjective symptoms. This is one of the many reasons why home peak flow measurement can be particularly valuable in controlling treatment in asthma.

Short courses of corticosteroids in the management of asthma should consist of oral prednisolone given in a dose of 30–40 mg orally daily[15]. This dose should be continued for seven to fourteen days, the exact length being judged by the response rate. With such short courses of oral steroids, there is no reason to tail down slowly, although this sometimes may be advisable in patients who have shown a deterioration soon after previous courses of steroids. This dose of corticosteroids can be given as a single dose in the morning.

There has been recent interest in the choice of corticosteroid, with some evidence that the responses may vary. However, these studies of drugs such as triamcinolone acetonide have been difficult to interpret because of the uncertainty in equivalence of doses. In general, prednisolone provides suitable therapy with easily adaptable dose formulations.

Few side-effects are associated with this form of corticosteroid treatment. Indigestion may be seen and is less with enteric coated prednisolone. Some fluid retention and increase in blood pressure may occur, as may glycosuria or deterioration of underlying diabetes. Much rarer side-effects are acute steroid myopathy and acute steroid psychosis.

Parenteral corticosteroids are sometimes necessary in acute severe asthma. They are really necessary only when there are likely to be problems with absorption of oral therapy, since there is little if any difference in the rate of onset of the response.

Inhaled corticosteroids. Inhaled beclomethasone dipropionate was introduced in 1972, and the alternative drugs betamethasone-17-valerate and budesonide have since been produced. These drugs have proved to be very effective in the management of asthma[16]. They have no benefit in acute attacks, but are used as long-term suppressive therapy. Great attention to patient education is necessary to ensure compliance with this form of inhaled therapy, where no immediate benefit is apparent. Once more, this can be helped by the demonstration of the benefit of a drug with home peak flow recording. There are few adverse effects of the use of inhaled steroids, but patients are often worried by the connotations of the term 'steroid'.

Initial worries concerned adrenal suppression. Biochemical evidence of effects on the hypothalamic–pituitary–adrenal axis have been demonstrated at doses about 1500–2000 μg daily of beclomethasone dipropionate. These effects have not been associated with clinical problems. The only other side-effects of inhaled steroids have related to changes within the oropharynx. There is a small incidence of oral candidiasis, and occasionally dysphonia may occur. Symptomatic oral candidiasis can be treated with nystatin pastilles or amphotericin lozenges, together with careful cleaning of any dentures. Further episodes may be prevented by reducing oropharyngeal impaction of the corticosteroid aerosol by use of a spacer device.

In the past inhaled corticosteroids have usually been given on a four times daily basis. In many cases, it is possible to manage on a twice daily regime. Most of the evidence suggests that this is probably slightly less effective than the four times daily administration, but this reduced effect is partially offset by better compliance with a twice daily dosage. Newer higher dose inhalers for steroids have made it easier to manipulate the dose of the inhaled drug. This should be matched to patients' needs in control of symptoms in the same way as oral therapy, rather than the routine administration of a fixed dose.

In patients with chronic airflow obstruction, inhaled corticosteroids can be used to follow on from a course of oral steroids which has been given to achieve maximum improvement in chronic airway narrowing.

Combined preparations

There is no longer any place for the numerous combined oral preparations which often contain ineffectively small doses of theophylline and outdated β-agonists such as ephedrine. However, many asthmatics do require more than one inhaled preparation and several combined inhalers are available. Duovent is a combination of fenoterol and ipratropium bromide which may sometimes be useful in subjects who have been shown to benefit from the addition of an anticholinergic agent to their β-agonist.

The other combined preparation is Ventide, which combines salbutamol with beclomethasone dipropionate. This suffers from the same problems as Intal Co. The fast bronchodilator action of salbutamol makes inappropriate use of the inhaled corticosteroid likely. A few patients may require stable regular therapy with both drugs and be reluctant to use more than one inhaler but, in general, it is better to keep these drugs, with their different actions, independent.

THE MANAGEMENT OF SPECIFIC SITUATIONS

There is a continuous spectrum in the severity of asthma from the subject who develops airway narrowing after exercise or exposure to an allergen, perhaps without ever noticing it, to the patient with a life-threatening severe attack. There may be a return to normal between episodes or there may be persistent obstruction with minor variation. We know now that even patients symptom-free between occasional attacks have continuing inflammatory damage in their airways, perpetuating their asthmatic tendency. With this spectrum of clinical types there are problems in making clear divisions with regard to treatment. In the following sections seven clinical situations will be considered:

(1) occasional asthma;
(2) exercise-induced asthma;
(3) persistent asthma;
(4) nocturnal asthma;
(5) acute severe asthma;
(6) asthma in childhood; and
(7) asthma in pregnancy.

Occasional Asthma

For the purposes of considering treatment a patient with occasional asthma will be regarded as one who has no airflow obstruction for most of the time and develops problems less than once a week. When symptoms occur more often than this, then some form of prophylactic treatment is usually indicated, but where the symptoms are occasional, symptomatic use of bronchodilators is sufficient. This will not be appropriate when the occasional attacks are severe. In that case suitable regular treatment will be justified to prevent these episodes. Opinions will obviously vary on the point at which regular treatment becomes justified. A simple rule of thumb might be that prophylactic therapy should be considered when:

(1) a mild episode requiring 2–4 puffs of a β-agonist occurs more than once a week; and
(2) a moderate episode requiring more than 4 puffs of a β-agonist occurs more than once a month.

The unsatisfactory part of these criteria lies in the subjective element. A more reliable decision can be made if a period of

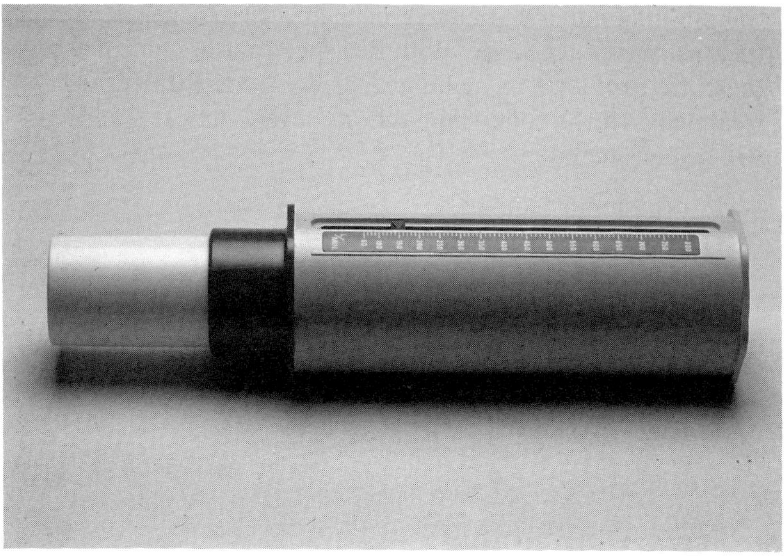

Figure 4.1 Peak flow meter

home peak flow recording is performed (Fig. 4.1). This will add an objective measurement; patients using only an occasional puff of β-agonist may have diurnal variation in peak flow and significant drops which they are not aware of or do not consider a sufficient indication for treatment. Such daily peak flow variability is related to airway reactivity and is likely to reflect the degree of continuing inflammation in the respiratory mucosa. There is now evidence that reactivity is reduced by appropriate specific treatment and, hopefully, this will reduce the inflammation, the likelihood of more severe attacks and the tendency to permanent airway damage.

Identifying Provocative Factors

The patient with occasional symptoms probably offers the best chance of identifying specific provocative factors. This should be considered in all asthmatic patients but becomes easier

Practical point

- a short period of home peak flow monitoring aids the choice of appropriate treatment even in patients with mild or infrequent symptoms.

when obvious exacerbations occur from a stable baseline. Specific external provoking factors are also more likely to be present in these patients. In obvious cases the patient will probably have made the association for him or herself. In other cases a careful history will reveal the provocative stimulus. Exposure may be minutes or many hours before the symptoms develop. When the onset is delayed the association may be more difficult to establish and requires a careful history. When an occupational element is likely, peak flow recording at home and at work should be performed[17]. When some dietary factor seems probable, then an accurate food diary often helps to bring it to light. When there is a suspicion of the involvement of some provocative factor, skin prick tests may help. If the history suggests acute precipitation the appropriate skin test will nearly always be positive. Occasionally, provocation tests are helpful but they should be performed only under supervision in experienced laboratories.

The purpose of identifying provocative factors lies mainly in the hope that subsequent avoidance will help in asthma control and reduce the need for medication. Despite the development of safe effective treatments which control most asthmatics, a reasonable search should always be made for provocative factors, and a careful history should be taken.

Practical point

- a careful history should always be taken to identify provocative factors for asthma.

Bronchodilator Treatment

If occasional episodes of asthma cannot be prevented by avoiding contact with provoking agents, then pharmacological treatment will be necessary. The usual way to deal with occasional mild wheezing is to use an inhaled bronchodilator as necessary. As mentioned earlier, frequent use implies that some other suppressive treatment should be used. Oral bronchodilators are too slow in their onset of action to have a place in this type of therapy. Oral β-agonists develop their effect over one to two hours, while inhaled treatment is beginning to work within five minutes and achieves its maximum effect in 15 to 30 minutes[2].

Even mild asthmatics may develop a more severe acute attack at some time. They must be educated to recognize the severity of such an attack and the need to seek further help, and they must know exactly how to find such help, taking higher doses of their bronchodilators while this is being obtained.

In most cases the choice of inhaled treatment will be a β-agonist rather than an anticholinergic agent. The onset of action is quicker and the response is often better. There is little to choose between the available β-agonists, and a more important consideration is the type of inhaler device.

Delivery of inhaled therapy

1. Metered dose inhalers. The majority of patients can be taught to use a metered dose inhaler efficiently. This should be demonstrated by the prescribing doctor and then the patient's own technique should be evaluated. Even if this seems to have been learnt, the technique should be regularly checked on subsequent visits. The important points in the administration of a metered dose inhaler are:

(1) shake the canister;
(2) take off the cap;
(3) breathe out;

(4) actuate the inhaler towards the start of a full slow, deep inspiration; and
(5) hold the breath at full inspiration for ten seconds.

Studies of the penetration of aerosol and the effects show that the initial expiration and the timing of the actuation may not be very important, and that better results may be obtained with the inhaler two inches from an open mouth. However, these details are more difficult to teach and, in practice, actuation at the beginning of a full inhalation is easiest for the patient to understand. Even with optimal technique most of the aerosol delivered impacts in the oropharynx and only about 9% reaches the respiratory tract.

2. Aids for metered dose inhalers. Around a quarter of asthmatic patients will be unable to use a metered dose inhaler efficiently. In some cases, such as patients with arthritis, this will be a problem of manipulation and the power to actuate the inhaler. These problems can be overcome by the use of devices which actuate the inhaler when squeezed (Figure 4.2).

3. Spacer devices. In most cases the problems are connected with difficulties in the coordination of the actuation and inspiration. Such problems are usually evident at the first attempts to use the inhaler. Two alternative approaches are to move to a metered dose inhaler with a spacer device, or to a dry powder system. Spacer devices come in various forms. A small extension tube may cope with minor degrees of hand–lung coordination and is collapsible enough to be carried round easily. The large spacer devices, such as the Nebuhaler and the Volumatic (Figure 4.3), take away any need to coordinate actuation and inhalation but are hardly easy to slip in a pocket or handbag. They have the advantage of reducing oropharyngeal drug deposition[18] and this helps patients who develop problems with oral candidiasis with inhaled corticosteroid therapy.

4. Dry powder systems. The alternative device is the dry powder rotacap system available for β-agonists and corticosteroids. Some patients find inhalation of the dry powder

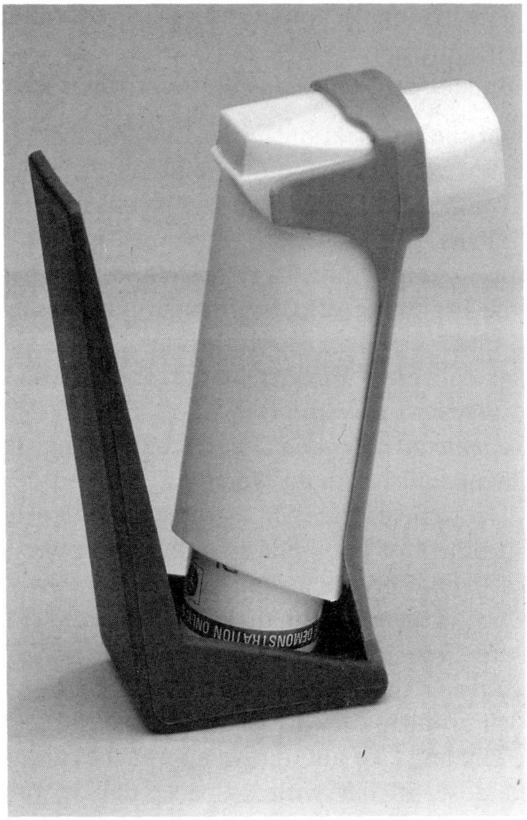

Figure 4.2 Metered dose inhaler for arthritic patient

irritates and induces coughing, but in most cases these systems provide a satisfactory alternative to metered dose inhalers. As with the inhalers patients should be taught carefully how to use the dry powder systems:

(1) push in the capsule, clear end first, until the outer end is level with the outside of the rotahaler;
(2) hold the rotahaler horizontal;
(3) twist the barrel fully in one direction and back;
(4) breathe out, place the mouthpiece between the teeth with the head tilted back;

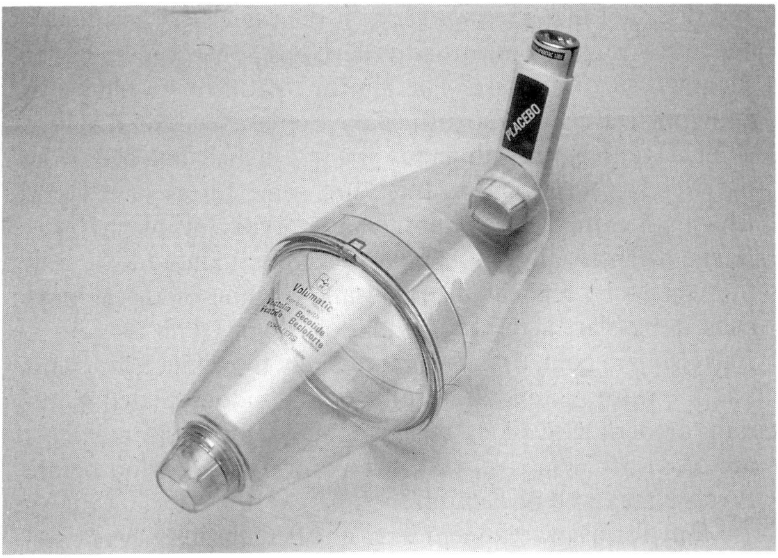

Figure 4.3 Large spacer device

(5) breathe in fully and quickly; and
(6) hold your breath for ten seconds.

Nebulizers would not be appropriate for this group with occasional asthma and are considered under chronic asthma and acute severe asthma.

When there are situations which are known to provoke asthma but which are unavoidable, then prophylactic bronchodilator therapy may be appropriate. This applies particularly to exercise-induced asthma.

Exercise-induced asthma

Exercise is a common provocative factor for asthma. When used as a specific challenge procedure around 75% of asthmatics will respond with a drop in FEV_1 of more than 10%. This wheezing is brought on by about six minutes of exercise and does not increase in severity if the exercise is prolonged. The airway narrowing usually develops some minutes after such a bout of exercise. The aim of treatment should be to allow the asthmatic patient to take exercise as desired. There is an advantage in asthmatics staying fit and not becoming overweight. Nevertheless, there are some forms of exercise which are more likely than others to provoke problems[19].

The mechanism of induction of exercise-induced asthma is thought to be related to drying and cooling of the airways caused by the increased ventilation involved in exercise[20]. Exercising in cold, dry air is more likely to produce problems and the warm, humid atmosphere of an indoor heated swimming pool is least likely to give trouble. Short sprint events are often problem free, and a gentle warm-up period before exercise may well be helpful.

Many forms of treatment have an effect in preventing exercise-induced asthma, and β-agonists are effective in reversing the effects once they occur. Occasional patients, mainly children, have a mild, late response with asthma developing some hours after exercise. Beta-agonists are the most effective prophylactic therapy. They should be given by inhalation 30 minutes before exercise. This form of therapy is allowed by most international sports authorities. Sodium cromoglycate is also effective even in this single dose prophylactic form. A few patients fail to respond to β-agonists or cromoglycate alone and need a combination of the two. Theophyllines may also work. Anticholinergic agents such as ipratropium bromide have a variable effect, being completely suppressive in some patients but ineffective in others. Prophylactic therapy with inhaled corticosteroids may also work, but only when given long term rather than as a single administration before exertion.

Practical point

- Beta-agonists are the most effective prophylactic agent for exercise-induced asthma.

Persistent Asthma

Persistent asthma may be of any severity. When there is persistent, mild asthma an approach is to give regular bronchodilator therapy. While this may be effective therapy, it does not affect the underlying bronchial hyper-reactivity. The inflammatory changes in the airway wall continue and this may lead to long-term damage and the continuation of the asthmatic state. These thoughts have led to an increase in the use of other prophylactic therapy such as sodium cromoglycate, inhaled corticosteroids and nedocromil, where there is some evidence that continued use decreases airway reactivity.

Mild Persistent Asthma

For mild persistent asthma the recommended treatment is to begin one of the agents mentioned above with the use of inhaled bronchodilators in addition. In young patients sodium cromoglycate is an appropriate first choice, since it is so free of any adverse effects and is often helpful. With the use of these agents education of the patient is essential, since the introduction of a drug such as sodium cromoglycate changes the philosophy of therapy from 'on demand' to regular therapy. It is not usually difficult to persuade an asthmatic to take an inhaled β-agonist when wheezing develops, since its effect is evident within minutes. It may be harder to persuade a patient to take an inhaler regularly when he is symptom-free, which is the aim of regular asthmatic therapy. Such education is more effective when it is supported by convincing objective data such as peak flow charts or symptom diaries.

Sodium cromoglycate therapy should be started at a dose of one spincap four times a day, or two puffs of the 5 mg inhaler four times a day. Treatment should continue at this dose for at least one month. If the dry powder of the spincap produces irritation or coughing it is best to move to a metered dose inhaler. If coordination is a problem and a dry powder system is necessary, then use of a β-agonist ten minutes earlier will usually avoid the problems.

At the end of the first month's treatment, an attempt should be made to evaluate the effect of the sodium cromoglycate. If the asthma has been rather variable this may be too early and the treatment may need to continue for another month before reassessment.

In other cases the response to the sodium cromoglycate may be evident by the end of the first month. If it is effective, then it should be continued in the same dose for three to six months. Subsequently, attempts can be made to reduce the dose, particularly to reduce the frequency of dosing to a more convenient regime. If the asthma is completely suppressed and need for additional bronchodilator therapy removed, then at some time a decision must be made about continuation of therapy. A reasonable programme is to reduce therapy to one spincap or two 5 mg puffs twice a day, and after six to twelve months to try to stop treatment. Earlier discontinuation of therapy is likely to be ineffective.

When the sodium cromoglycate appears to be ineffective after a reasonable time in a compliant patient, then the next step is to switch to inhaled corticosteroid therapy. In patients over 30 years of age the chances of responding initially to sodium cromoglycate are fewer and there is a reasonable argument for using inhaled corticosteroids in the first place. This avoids any problems of losing the patient's confidence with a failed trial of prophylactic therapy. Alternatively, it is a situation where the newer drug nedocromil sodium may have a place. There seems to be no benefit in combining sodium cromoglycate and inhaled corticosteroids but nedocromil and corticosteroids may be a useful combination.

Inhaled corticosteroids are given as a trial in the same way as sodium cromoglycate, monitoring the response by symptoms, bronchodilator use and peak flow rate if possible. In mild asthma it is satisfactory to begin treatment with twice daily therapy, such as 200–400 μg of beclomethasone dipropionate twice daily. At the end of a month this treatment is assessed. If the response is inadequate then the dose should be increased. At doses of 2000 μg effects on biochemical tests of the hypothalamo–pituitary–adrenal axis can be demonstrated[21]. The mild adrenal suppression at these high doses has to be weighed against the effects of alternative treatments such as oral corticosteroids.

If the above treatments in combination with bronchodilator therapy as necessary are ineffective, then it is unlikely that the picture is that of mild persistent asthma, and more substantial therapy will be necessary.

Persistent Moderate or Severe Asthma

The approach to persistent asthma, which is not controlled by sodium cromoglycate or inhaled corticosteroids, differs in that continuous administration of bronchodilators is likely to be necessary since the airflow obstruction is persistent in addition to suppressive therapy with sodium cromoglycate or inhaled corticosteroids. In order to obtain optimal bronchodilatation a higher dose or a combination of bronchodilators may be appropriate.

The suppressive therapy will usually consist of the most effective dose of inhaled corticosteroids. This should be judged by the effect obtained up to a daily dose equivalent to 1600 or 2000 μg of beclomethasone dipropionate. Even if it is necessary to go onto oral corticosteroids to achieve adequate control, the inhaled drugs should be continued to minimize the dose of oral therapy.

Before resorting to continuous oral corticosteroids an alternative approach of intermittent courses should be tried. It is well recognized that short courses of corticosteroids are effective in deteriorating asthma and in acute attacks. Such courses, 30–40 mg of prednisolone for two weeks, often have a prolonged effect in persistent, moderate asthma. They may produce significant improvement, which then leaves a sustained effect for several months, when a further course may be necessary. A regime such as this, with three or four courses a year and continuous inhaled corticosteroids can result in a lower overall steroid dose and far less adrenal suppression than continuous low dose oral therapy.

When it is felt essential to give continuous oral corticosteroids, they should be given as alternate day therapy in the morning when possible. This is usually effective unless the equivalent daily dose rises above 10 mg prednisolone.

With regard to continuous bronchodilator therapy in persistent asthma, inhaled therapy is still in general preferable to oral treatment because of the lower incidence of adverse effects. In many cases adequate doses of β-agonists are sufficient. Alternative therapy needs to be sought when:

(1) the β-agonists effect is inadequate;
(2) side effects are troublesome; or
(3) the dose required needs an inconvenient number of inhalations.

When the response to β-agonists is inadequate, the options are to increase the dose or to add a second bronchodilator agent. There is a wide range of dose responses among asthmatic patients and in some cases it is difficult to give the dose required by conventional inhaled therapy. This is one circumstance where nebulizer therapy should be considered.

If the response to high dose β-agonist therapy is still inadequate, or adverse effects occur, then combined therapy is indicated. A certain number of patients with persistent airflow obstruction, perhaps a quarter or a third, have a further response to anticholinergic agents above their maximal β-agonist response. This combination is, therefore, worth attempting. There is little evidence that theophyllines add to the maximal β-agonist effect, but they provide a means of restricting the β-agonist dose by an additive effect at lower doses.

When anticholinergic agents are to be used in addition with β-agonists, the existence of some further response should be established by objective measurements. The same applies to the addition of theophylline therapy, when the serum level should also be checked and the dose adjusted to give a level well within the therapeutic range[9]. Once on theophylline a watch must be kept on additional therapy to avoid drug interactions (Table 4.3).

Nebulizer Therapy

The three main uses for nebulizers in asthma[4] are to overcome difficulties in inhalation technique, to provide high dose regular therapy and to treat acute severe attacks.

The first indication applies mainly to children who, though too young to use metered dose inhalers and dry powder systems, can be controlled on regular sodium cromoglycate, corticosteroids or β-agonists by way of a nebulizer. The third group is the most worrying, since the home use of nebulizers brings the potential danger of patients staying at home and treating themselves when they need hospital or other care. This will be dealt with in the section on acute severe asthma.

In persistent moderate asthma the use of nebulizers is generally the second option above, to provide regular high dose therapy with β-agonists or anticholinergic agents. In order to qualify for a home nebulizer for this purpose, the patient must show that such high dose therapy is necessary, i.e. objective measurements must demonstrate that the response to 2.5 mg or 5 mg by nebulizer is significantly better than four or six puffs of metered dose inhaler.

Two main types of nebulizer are available. Most widely used is the jet nebulizer driven by a source of compressed air or oxygen. In acute severe asthma the driving source should be oxygen, if possible, but for general use an air compressor is satisfactory. This should provide a flow rate of greater than 4 l/min. The nebulizer chamber should be filled with 3–4 ml of fluid, the drug diluted with isotonic saline. The alternative nebulizer is the ultrasonic type where the solution is nebulized by vibration of piezo-electric crystal. These devices are more expensive than the most jet nebulizers run by air compressors. A third alternative is the foot pump driven jet nebulizer but this is more suitable for occasional emergency use rather than regular therapy (Fig. 4.4).

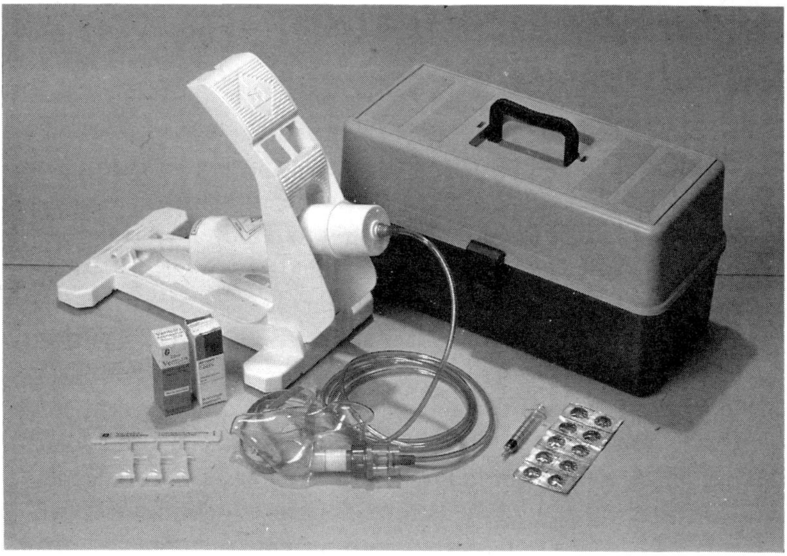

Figure 4.4 Foot pump driven jet nebulizer

If a patient is relying on a nebulizer for regular bronchodilator therapy, then a backup and maintenance service should exist to check the nebulizer regularly and provide a substitute if the machine breaks down. Such services are best organized through the local chest clinic. To avoid problems it is advisable for patients not to obtain their own machines outside such a service. They should certainly not be available without the sanction of a doctor.

Practical point

Stepped regime for persistent moderate asthma

1. High dose inhaled corticosteroids
2. Regular bronchodilator therapy
3. Maximize bronchodilator response by high dose or combination therapy
4. Occasional doses of oral corticosteroids
5. Regular alternate day oral corticosteroids.

Nocturnal Asthma

Nocturnal wheezing and cough are common symptoms in asthmatics. In normal subjects there is a small diurnal variation in airway calibre[22]. The amplification of this rhythm in asthmatic subjects can be troublesome to treat. The diurnal variation in asthmatics is related to bronchial hyper-responsiveness. Therefore, the first approach to treatment should be to treat the general hyper-responsiveness with drugs such as inhaled corticosteroids, rather than concentrate simply on the matching of treatment to night-time symptoms.

However, when regular daily treatment fails to relieve the nocturnal asthma, then long-acting nightly bronchodilators may be necessary. Inhaled bronchodilators taken at bedtime do not last long enough to provide protection and oral slow-release preparations are more suitable. Slow release theophylline and slow release β-agonist preparations seem to be effective. They can be given as a single night-time dose and have been shown to improve sleep, reduce nocturnal inhaler use and reduce diurnal variation in peak flow rate.

The pharmacokinetics of theophylline vary between day and night; a large dose may be necessary to produce an adequate effect, but side-effects are not common with the patient lying down at night. The blood level of theophylline should be checked on an early morning blood sample.

Acute Severe Asthma

The continuing death rate from acute asthma shows the importance of the appropriate treatment of this condition. The evidence shows that the majority of the problems are related to inadequate assessment and treatment of acute asthma[14]. The first stage is to appreciate the severity of an attack of asthma. Pointers to a severe attack are:

(1) pulse rate above 110/minute;
(2) respiratory rate above 25/minute;
(3) inability to talk in sentences;
(4) peak flow below 100/minute;
(5) cyanosis; and
(6) use of accessory muscles to breathe.

A patient who shows one or more of the above features is likely to need admission to hospital for treatment. The worsening of an attack of asthma can often be abated at an earlier stage by the use of a timely course of oral corticosteroids[15]. Once the decision to admit a patient to hospital has been made, the general practitioner should administer a corticosteroid as intravenous hydrocortisone or oral prednisolone, and a β-stimulant by nebulizer or subcutaneous route. The important elements to consider in the treatment of acute severe asthma are discussed below.

Bronchodilator Therapy

There appears to be no advantage in using parenteral β-agonists over nebulized drugs, and nebulized β-agonists work as well or better than intravenous aminophylline. Therefore, the initial bronchodilator drug of choice is nebulized salbutamol or terbutaline. Salbutamol should be given as an initial dose of 5 mg made up to 4 ml with normal saline, and the nebulizer driven by oxygen. If the patient has a history of ischaemic heart disease or arrhythmias then the dose should be restricted to 2.5 mg. Should this first nebulization produce no response in 30 minutes, it should be repeated at double the initial dose.

When the second dose also fails to give significant benefit, then an alternative bronchodilator and/or alternative route will need to be considered. This may be the addition of nebulized ipratropium bromide, or the use of intravenous therapy in the form of a β-agonist, or aminophylline. If the response is adequate, nebulized therapy should be continued every three to four hours.

If aminophylline is used, account should be taken of previous oral therapy is selecting the dose. If patients on oral therapy are known to have therapeutic blood levels from previous or emergency results, then no leading dose is necessary and a continuous infusion of around 0.5 mg/kg/hr can be used. When no level is available, a compromise of halving the loading dose from 5 mg/kg to 2.5 mg/kg seems to be reasonable and is rarely associated with problems. The loading dose of intravenous aminophylline should, of course, be given slowly and steadily over 15 to 20 minutes.

The response to treatment can be judged by the clinical state of the patient. Heart rate, respiratory rate, peak flow and the degree of paradox in the blood pressure are used to assess the response to treatment. Many of the severe problems and some of the asthma deaths occur several days after the acute admission, when diurnal variation is returning with big morning dips and therapy is being withdrawn. Throughout the acute episode it is important to monitor response to the treatment given, and to keep a careful watch on the patient. Treatment with steroids and high dose bronchodilators should not be reduced just because daytime peak flow is beginning to improve; they should be continued to obtain good, sustained improvement.

Corticosteroids

Corticosteroids are a vital part of the management of acute episodes. They take some hours to develop their beneficial effect, so that treatment of significant exacerbations should begin early. Unless the attack is very severe oral prednisolone provides satisfactory therapy and there is no advantage in using parenteral hydrocortisone[23]. In fact hydrocortisone produces occasional adverse effects in asthmatics. Prednisolone should be given in a dose of 60 mg initially, followed by 40 mg daily. If hydrocortisone is used, the drug should be 200 mg intravenously six-hourly. This can be converted to prednisolone after the first 24 or 48 hours.

Prednisolone should be continued for 10–14 days in a dose of 30 or 40 mg, when it can be stopped abruptly provided a complete response appears to have been obtained. This is based on reaching predicted lung function or the patient's previous best levels. It is generally judged on peak flow or spirometry measurements, but full return to normal based on lung volumes and airflow at low lung volumes may take longer to return to normal. There are few significant adverse effects from such brief courses of corticosteroids and they should not be stopped too soon. Inadequate treatment of the acute episode is likely to lead to a premature return of problems.

Practical point

- oral prednisolone is adequate for acute episodes of asthma unless the attack is severe enough to compromise cardiac output and affect absorption.

Oxygen

The typical blood gas changes in acute severe asthma are hypoxia and hypocapnia. Supplementing inspired oxygen is an important part of the management. Hypercapnia is an unusual finding which develops when the patient is becoming exhausted and is generally in urgent need of ventilatory support. Hypercapnia is not induced by supplemental inspired oxygen, which can be given freely. In older patients, with chronic airflow obstruction from chronic bronchitis and emphysema, increasing the inspired oxygen can worsen hypercapnia, so careful control of the oxygen concentration is necessary[24]. However, it is usually easy to recognize such patients from their age and history.

In hypoxic patients nebulizers should be driven by oxygen rather than air. There is a largely theoretical possibility that bronchodilators may worsen hypoxia but it is more important that those patients who need supplemental oxygen should not have it discontinued for the ten to fifteen minutes necessary for nebulization.

Fluid

Patients in an acute attack of asthma are likely to become dehydrated because of increased fluid loss associated with increased ventilation and decreased oral input because of breathlessness. This will need to be made up with intravenous fluids, a reasonable volume being 3 l in the first 24 hours.

Potassium

A number of factors contribute to the development of hypokalaemia in acute severe asthma. The corticosteroids, β-agonists and methylxanthines all contribute in addition to the effects of hyperventilation itself. Potassium levels should be checked and potassium added to the intravenous fluid as appropriate.

Antibiotics

Antibiotics are often given as a routine part of the treatment of acute asthma. There is no evidence that this approach is warranted. Where there is an infectious element precipitating the attack it is almost always viral. The problem comes in identifying the patient who does have a bacterial infection. Fever and leukocytosis are common findings in acute asthma and purulent sputum may just reflect a prominent eosinophilia.

A suitable compromise is to use an appropriate antibiotic such as amoxycillin or erythromycin when fever is high or sputum obviously purulent.

Ventilation

Occasionally patients present too quickly or too late to respond to the above therapy so that they deteriorate to a stage where assisted ventilation is necessary. The decision to ventilate is based mainly on the clinical status supplemented by blood gas analysis. The outcome of ventilation is good if it is undertaken as an elective measure, but poor if respiratory arrest is the indication. Ventilation of asthmatic patients presents problems because of the high pressures required and the time needed for passive expiration to occur. It is a process which requires experienced anaesthetic expertise. Nebulized drugs can be continued during ventilation.

Other measures

There is no evidence that mucolytic agents are of any use. Airway hydration is probably useful particularly during ventilation, but this is provided by the nebulized therapy.

Sedation is never indicated in acute severe asthma unless ventilation is being taken over. Distress is generally related to dyspnoea and hypoxia.

Breathing exercises assiduously learnt while in remission are difficult to maintain during an acute attack. Physiotherapy has little part to play except to help cough up plugs of sputum if these are troublesome. However, physiotherapists are often the most experienced staff in the management of nebulizer therapy.

Occasionally, once a patient has been ventilated and hypoxia and high airway pressures are maintained despite appropriate therapy, then fibreoptic bronchoscopy and lung lavage may help to remove tenacious plugs from the airways. This requires careful consideration because hypoxia is likely to worsen during and for a short time after bronchoscopy.

After the Acute Attack

Patients are vulnerable in the days after an acute attack. Airway lability is usually high with a large diurnal variation in airway calibre. The intensive therapy used to overcome the initial problems must not be discontinued too soon.

The occurrence of an acute attack should always stimulate a review of routine therapy, the measures taken during the initial deterioration, and the acute episode. Plans must be made to try to achieve control which avoids admission to hospital in the future.

Asthma in Childhood

Education is even more important and more challenging in childhood asthma than adult asthma, since the education has to involve the parents and teachers as well as the patient. A number of teaching aids in the form of books, comics and visual aids are now available to help in this essential field. The aim should be to encourage as normal a lifestyle as possible, using suitable therapy to allow participation in sports and other activities.

Overall the approaches to the types of asthma are similar in children to those discussed in adults[25]. Differences relate to the practicalities of using inhaled drugs in children, the greater likelihood of response to sodium cromoglycate, and worries about the effects of corticosteroid treatment and uncontrolled asthma itself on growth.

Hyposensitization and Antigen Avoidance

Some studies suggest that hyposensitization with dust mite extracts is of some benefit but the dangers of this form of therapy mean that, currently, it is reserved for patients with established mite allergy poorly controlled by routine therapy. It should be carried out only under close observation, with resuscitation facilities immediately available.

Antigen avoidance is also disappointing unless the patient is moved to a dust-free environment. It does not seem to be practical to achieve adequate reduction in mite numbers in the normal home environment. Future developments in mite eradication may change this picture.

The Inhalation Route in Children

For the reasons discussed in the adult section, inhaled treatment is nearly always preferable to oral therapy. Under four years of age children are unable to perform an adequate deep inspiration so that treatment must be with a nebulizer or, occasionally, a nebuhaler. From the age of four onwards, other inhaled therapy is usually possible with dry powder inhalers. Metered dose inhalers are more difficult in younger children but can be tried over the age of six or seven. When inhaled therapy is not achievable, oral theophylline or β-stimulants may be necessary.

Asthma in Infancy

Under the age of 18 months the responses to bronchodilators are disappointing. There are reports of paradoxical bronchoconstriction in response to nebulized salbutamol. This should always be given under close supervision in the first instance. Nebulized ipratropium bromide may be effective in infants but moderate wheezing is primarily treated with oxygen and hydration.

Treatment of Chronic Asthma in Children

In children with asthma who need more than occasional bronchodilators inhaled sodium cromoglycate should generally be the first approach because of the lack of side-effects. If an adequate one or two month trial of sodium cromoglycate with bronchodilators fails to achieve control, then inhaled corticosteroids should be used. If possible the dose should be kept below 1000 μg beclomethasone dipropionate, although even at this dose it may be possible to detect an effect on the hypothalamo–pituitary–adrenal axis in children[26]. However, growth does not appear to be affected and the adverse effects of uncontrolled asthma are more of a problem than any minor biochemical effects of inhaled corticosteroids.

Occasionally it is necessary to use oral corticosteroids long term, but this should be undertaken only when other aggressive inhaled therapy has failed. Oral corticosteroids should be given as a single dose on alternate days.

Acute Severe Asthma

In the same way as adults, children and their parents must have a clear idea of exactly what to do if there is an exacerbation of asthma. This education will also need to be extended to school teachers.

Children under three years of age are difficult to assess, and if there are any doubts treatment should err on the side of caution, using corticosteroids, nebulized β-agonists and hospital admission. Over the age of 18 months, the treatment of a severe attack of asthma follows that in adults, with suitable adjustment in dosages of corticosteroids (hydrocortisone 4 mg/kg 6-hourly). As in adults, sustained improvement should be ensured before treatment is reduced and careful supervision relaxed.

Asthma in pregnancy

Pregnancy has a variable effect on the control of asthma. Severe asthma tends to worsen. Overall, around 50% of asthmatics show little change, 30% improve and 20% worsen. The pattern is usually consistent in subsequent pregnancies.

Selective β-agonists are safe and effective but adrenaline, ephedrine and isoprenaline should be avoided. Theophyllines cross the placenta and enter breast milk. They may produce irritability in newborn and breast fed infants but no long-term effects are known. Inhaled sodium cromoglycate is safe in pregnancy.

Inhaled corticosteroids appear to be safe. It has been suggested that oral steroids are associated with cleft palate and still births but the risks, if any, seem to be very small. They are less than the problems of uncontrolled asthma, and prednisolone should be used for deteriorating asthma when necessary.

REFERENCES

1. Barnes, P. J., Karliner, J. S. and Dollery, C. T. (1980). Human lung adrenoceptors studied by radioligand binding. *Clin. Sci.*, **58,** 457–61
2. Webb, J., Rees, J. and Clark, T. J. H. (1982). A comparison of the effects of different methods of administration of beta$_2$-sympathomimetics in patients with asthma. *Br. J. Dis. Chest,* **76,** 351–7
3. Neville, E., Corris, P. A., Vivian, J., Nariman, S. and Gibson, G. J. (1982). Nebulised salbutamol and angina. *Br. Med. J.,* **285,** 796–7
4. Cochrane, G. M., Prior, J. G., Rees, P. J. (1985). Home nebulisers in the management of airflow limitation. *Br. Med. J.,* **290,** 1608–9
5. Engelhardt, A. and Klupp, H. (1975). The pharmacology and toxicology of a new tropane alkaloid derivative. *Postgrad. Med. J.,* **51** (Suppl 7), 82
6. Ward, M. J., Fentem, P. H., Roderick-Smith, W. H., and Davies D. (1981). Ipratropium bromide in acute asthma. *Br. Med. J.,* **282,** 598–600
7. Nadel, J. A. (1984). Adoration of the vagi. *N. Eng. J. Med.,* **311,** 463–4
8. Rafferty, P., Beasley, R., Howarth, P. H., Mann, J. S. and Holgate, S. T. (1986). Bronchoconstriction induced by nebulised ipratropium bromide: relation to the bromide ion. *Br. Med. J.,* **293,** 1538–9
9. Weinberger, M. and Hendeles, L. (1983). Use of theophylline for asthma. In: Clark, T. J. H. and Godfrey, S. (eds) *Asthma,* 2nd Edition (London, Chapman and Hall)

10. Woodcock, A. A., Johnson, M. A. and Geddes, D. M. (1983). Theophylline prescribing, serum concentrations and toxicity. *Lancet,* **2,** 610–2
11. Barnes, P., Neville, L., Greening, A. P., Timms, J. and Poole, G. N. (1982). Single dose slow release aminophylline at night prevents nocturnal asthma. *Lancet,* **1,** 299–301
12. Godfrey, S. and Konig, P. (1976). Inhibition of exercise induced asthma by different pharmacological pathways. *Thorax,* **31,** 137
13. Adinoff, A. D. and Hollester, J. R. (1983). Steroid-induced fractures and bone loss in patients with asthma. *N. Eng. J. Med.,* **309,** 265–8
14. British Thoracic Association. (1982). Death from asthma in two regions of England. *Br. Med. J.,* **285,** 1251–5
15. Webb, J. R. (1986). Dose response of patients to oral corticosteroid treatment during exacerbations of asthma. *Br. Med. J.,* **292,** 1045–7
16. Clark, T. J. H. (Ed). (1983). *Steroids in Asthma.* (Auckland, ADIS Press)
17. Parkes, W. R. (1982). *Occupational Lung Disorders.* pp. 415–53 (London, Butterworth & Co)
18. Newman, S. P. (1983). Deposition and effects of inhalation aerosols. (Lund, Astra)
19. Silverman, M. and Anderson, S. D. (1972). Standardization of exercise tests in asthmatic children. *Arch. Dis. Child.* **47,** 882–9
20. Anderson, S. D. (1984). Is there a unifying hypothesis for exercise-induced asthma? *J. Allergy. Clin. Immunol.,* **73,** 660–5
21. Choo-Kang, Y. F. J., Cooper, J. E. and Grany, I. W. B. (1972). Beclomethasone dipropionate by inhalation in the treatment of airway obstruction. *Br. J. Dis. Chest.,* **66,** 101
22. Hetzel, M. R. and Clark, T. J. H. (1980). Comparison of normal and asthmatic circadian rhythms in peak expiratory flow rate. *Thorax,* **35,** 732–8
23. Harrison, B. D. W., Stokes, T. C., Hart, G. J., Vaughan, D. A., Ali, N. J. and Robinson, A. A. (1986). Need for intravenous hydrocortisone in addition to oral prednisolone in patients admitted to hospital with severe asthma without ventilatory failure. *Lancet,* **1,** 781–4
24. Gunawardena, K. A., Patel, B., Campbell, I. A., Macdonald, J. B. and Smith, A. P. (1984). Oxygen as a driving gas for nebulizers: safe or dangerous? *Br. Med. J.,* **288,** 272–4
25. Price, J. (1984). Asthma in childhood. *Br. Med. J.,* **288,** 1666–8
26. Law, M., Marchant, J. L., Honour, J. W., Preece, M. A. and Warner, J. O. (1986). Nocturnal adrenal suppression in asthmatic children taking inhaled beclomethasone dipropionate. *Lancet,* **1,** 942–4

5

THE FUTURE

INTRODUCTION

At present, much asthma still goes unrecognized in general practice. Even though doctors have been encouraged to use this diagnostic label more openly, many patients with coughing, wheezing and shortness of breath are undiagnosed when referred to hospital outpatient clinics. This applies particularly to the very young and to the elderly, whereas asthma appears to be more readily appreciated in young adults. There must be significantly more unrecognized asthma in the community in patients whose symptoms are less severe, or who are more stoical.

Patients are often found to have asthma which is only partially reversible, or so severe as to be almost irreversible. Does this imply a failure to treat earlier in the disease process? Large numbers of patients arrive at outpatient clinics quite unable to use the inhalers which they have been prescribed, sometimes for years, and will say when questioned that no-one ever showed them or checked their technique. Inhaled steroids are still underused in asthma, with too much reliance being placed on bronchodilator therapy alone and with long-acting theophylline or aminophylline preparations being added in when salbutamol fails. Patients still believe that they are allergic to all forms of salbutamol because the little pink tablets make them shake, and sometimes their general practitioners seem to support them in this belief.

Tragically, between 1500 and 2000 people still die from asthma in England and Wales each year (see Chapter 2) and all the surveys that have been carried out in this sensitive area have shown management in the final attack to have been less than ideal in the majority of cases. Against this background, many patients are turning to alternative medicine for help, and to allergy clinics of varying degrees of respectability in order to find a cure for their asthma which will rid them of the need to take medication. Treatments of no proven benefit are widely used, while treatments of proven efficacy and safety are grossly underused.

Asthma management in the future will require not only the development of new drugs and new techniques, but more immediately, the greater use of existing knowledge. The present for some doctors still lies in the future for others. This chapter will highlight some of the developments which I would like to see over the next few years, first of all on the basis of current knowledge, and then with the possibility of new advances in our understanding of asthma.

THE FUTURE: APPLYING CURRENT KNOWLEDGE

Reducing Morbidity: Making the Diagnosis

The first step in reducing asthma morbidity lies in recognizing the condition so that there is at least a possibility of correct treatment being applied. Any patient who has recurrent episodes of coughing or wheezing and breathlessness should be considered as a possible asthmatic. If the patient is a child, the presence of an atopic disorder in a parent or sibling strengthens the case for asthma, and the next step depends on the child's age. If very young, then measurement of peak flow rate (PFR) will not be possible and a trial of sodium cromoglycate or inhaled steroid should be considered – disappearance of symptoms over a few weeks, with no recurrence, is diagnostic of asthma. A trial of prednisolone may be indicated even in small children. Older children may be able to measure PFR before and after bronchodilator to show improvement, or before and after exercise-induced asthma[1].

In older patients, the diagnosis of asthma may be more readily made, but some general practitioners feel that a history of smoking, even in the past, means that any breathlessness and wheeze must be due to chronic bronchitis. Asthma can occur for the first time at any age and even genuine chronic bronchitis may be complicated by an asthmatic component. Measurement of PFR can be invaluable. This is a point which has been made frequently over the past few years, and it is disappointing to see only a slow response in the majority of general practitioner colleagues. Attention to detail is important, and patients should be taught to put the mouthpiece of the peak flow meter well into the mouth to avoid an artificially-high blow from the use of the tongue[2]. Single measurements of PFR are rarely useful because asthma is, by definition, variable airflow obstruction, implying at least two different peak flow readings on different occasions. Remember too that peak flow rates may well be normal when the patient comes to the surgery even though at 4 a.m. the patient was woken by wheezing. Figure 5.1 is a record which a 65-year-old patient made with a peak flow meter over 14 days. He had been complaining of unpredictable breathlessness, and had only a moderately reduced peak flow rate when seen in the general practitioner's surgery. He was told that his problem was due to obesity and anxiety. Anxious he certainly was, and with good reason. The large diurnal variation in PFR can be clearly seen, with the lowest values in the early morning, when he was woken from sleep by a sensation of being unable to breathe. Figure 5.2 shows the peak flow chart of an elderly man who was breathless and tight in the chest especially in the morning. The marked morning dip characteristic of asthma is seen, which improves as prednisolone is added. He is now maintained on inhaled steroids perfectly well. The chart also shows

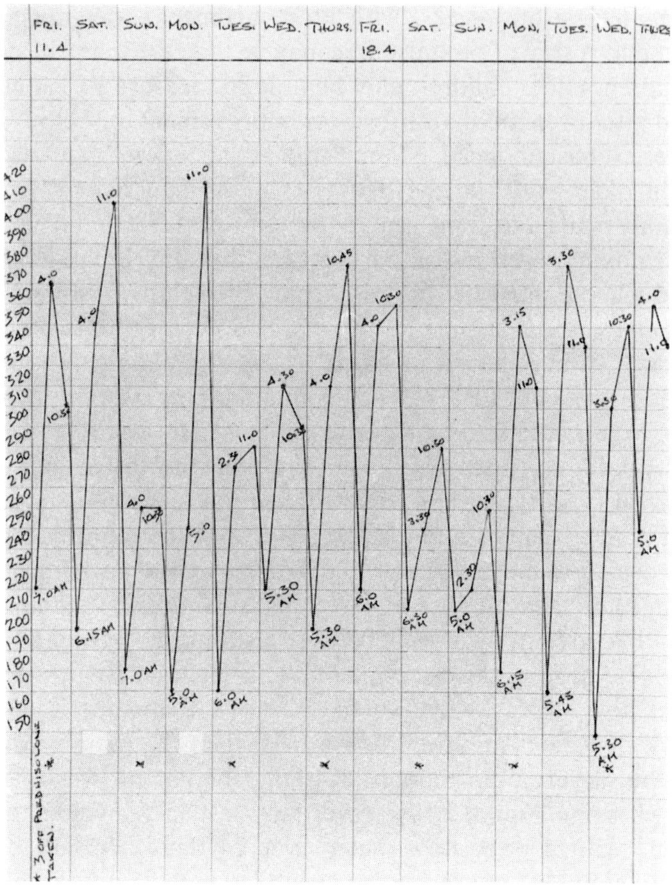

Figure 5.1 Peak flow chart kept at home by a man whose breathlessness had been ascribed to anxiety. His PFR showed enormous morning dips, often to half the afternoon level, even when he was taking a small dose of prednisolone regularly

how an afternoon or evening visit to the surgery would produce a misleadingly good PFR.

There is nothing difficult in the approach outlined above, and nothing which a general practitioner cannot do unaided. Hospital referral is of course necessary sometimes but the additional tests which can be done are few. More detailed

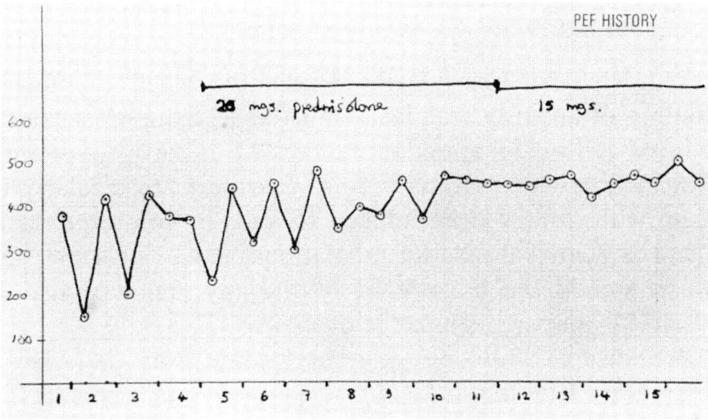

Figure 5.2 Peak flow chart (PFR on vertical axis, days on horizontal axis) from a patient with a rather non-specific story of difficulty in breathing. The morning dip, typical of uncontrolled asthma, gradually disappears on prednisolone

lung function tests may help in some cases where the airflow obstruction is chronic, where smoking may have played a part, and measurement of bronchial hyper-reactivity may assist diagnosis or management (see below).

Most general practitioners would not think twice about a trial of glyceryl trinitrate for a patient with chest pain but still seem reluctant to try corticosteroids for wheezing. The side-effects of a short course of steroids are likely to be far less than those of glyceryl trinitrate and the potential benefits of a correct diagnosis enormous. In the future, more doctors should be prepared to grasp the nettle in this way. Objective measurements are important and a small stock of peak flow meters to lend the patient is invaluable. There are some situations where either the doctor or the patient is reluctant to use oral steroids (e.g. active peptic ulcer, brittle diabetes) and a trial of high-dose inhaled steroids can be an effective substitute[3], provided of course that the patient can use the inhalational device correctly.

Reducing Morbidity: Morbidity at School

Recent work has clearly demonstrated the benefit to affected children of an early diagnosis of asthma[4]. Symptoms can be reduced and school attendance increased by early use of anti-asthma drugs; this means sodium cromoglycate regularly to begin with, followed by inhaled steroids in non-responders. There is nearly always an inhalational device of some sort which a child can use effectively and any prejudice against inhalers from parents must be overcome.

Prejudice of a different sort may come from the schools themselves. Children may not be allowed to take inhalers to school or keep them. Local paediatricians are usually able to give advice on this, and many teachers have now attended meetings organized by local branches of the Asthma Society. Awareness will be increased in the future.

Exercise-induced asthma is a particular problem for children at school, but there ought to be few children with asthma who cannot lead a normal life and take part in sport and games as much as they wish. Exercise-induced asthma can be prevented by prior administration of an inhaled β-agonist such as salbutamol or terbutaline, and it is desirable that children should have control over this themselves rather than having to approach an adult to allow them to use their inhaler. Some patients may require more than just two puffs (or equivalent) and should be told to experiment with a larger dose to see if this prevents their exercise-induced asthma[5]. There is now increasing evidence that regular inhaled steroids can reduce the bronchial hyper-reactivity which leads to exercise-induced asthma, and a greater awareness of this in the future should lead to reduced morbidity, in children particularly[6].

One further aspect of the treatment of asthma in children is the benefit which can come from exercise training[7]. The improvement in exercise capability and morale even in quite severe asthmatics can be striking. Less formally, asthmatic children (or adults) who experience exercise-induced asthma can be taught to warm up gradually before a period of hard exercise by doing very short bursts of exertion. These should be insufficient to bring on an attack of exercise-induced asthma, but may be enough to generate refractoriness to asthma following more prolonged exercise.

Reducing Morbidity: Older Patients

Children have a remarkable tolerance to drugs and paediatricians regularly prescribe drugs which, on a mg/kg basis, would be quite unacceptable to adults. In asthma, this applies to two oral drugs, the β-agonists such as salbutamol and terbutaline, and methylxanthines such as theophylline. Oral β-agonists are still widely prescribed for adults, and may cause tremor and palpitations, side-effects which may prejudice a patient (or some general practitioners) from trying an inhaled form of the same drug. Inhaled bronchodilators are more rapid and effective than their oral equivalents, at a much smaller dose, and consequently produce fewer side-effects. There is really a very limited place for oral β-agonists in treating adult asthma, a message which has been accepted by many general practitioners, but the corollary that inhaled bronchodilators should be given by some means or other is still not pursued actively enough. It is well-known that many asthmatics cannot use aerosols[8], but in practice too little time is spent on trying an alternative inhalational device such as a powder inhaler, spacer, Nebuhaler or Volumatic device. Other devices are available from the pharmaceutical companies who make the most commonly-used aerosols, so that patients with a good idea of how to use an aerosol, but with arthritic hands, can manage them successfully. It really is uncommon to find a patient who cannot take inhaled bronchodilators with the aid of one or other of the devices currently available, although this is not yet widely appreciated in general practice. Some adults are resistant to the very idea of inhalers, perhaps linked to the publicity associated with the increase in asthma deaths in the late 1960s (see Chapter 2). They can usually be reassured when the facts are explained to them.

While doctors who prescribe inhalers have the responsibility of checking that patients can use them, pharmacists who supply them are likely to become more involved. Pharmacy students are increasingly taught about the clinical applications of drugs, as the pharmacists' role changes with the diminishing need for old-fashioned pharmacy techniques. In the future, every patient who presents a prescription for an inhaler to a pharmacist should be asked if they had had this particular inhaler before, and if not, the pharmacist should check their ability to use it. I would consider it perfectly acceptable, indeed desirable, for the pharmacist then to inform a general practitioner of a patient's inability to use a particular device, and would hope that the general practitioner could then make constructive suggestions as to an alternative approach.

The other oral bronchodilator which is widely used and indeed increasing in popularity, is theophylline, either on its own or combined with ethylenediamine as aminophylline. The increased usage is due to the availability of slow-release formulations and heavy promotion from the pharmaceutical companies. Theophylline undoubtedly has a place in asthma management, but general practitioners at present have a limited understanding of its metabolism and interactions[9]. To use theophylline properly, serum levels should be checked as is widely done by primary care physicians in the USA. General practitioners in this country will have to become more familiar with the concept of therapeutic drug monitoring. Theophylline clearance in general decreases with age, which is why children (other than infants) can tolerate it quite well, and why elderly patients do not. Apart from this general factor, older patients tend to have more co-existing diseases and to be taking other drugs which may alter theophylline clearance . Anyone taking theophylline should be told of the dangers of taking extra tablets, and the need to tell doctors who may wish to give them emergency treatment that they are on a particular tablet. Perhaps in future all patients on theophylline therapy should carry a card, similar to a steroid card, indicating the dose of theophylline taken.

There are major benefits to be gained from using inhaled steroids, in terms of reduced morbidity from asthma and possibly reduced mortality (see below) and these compounds produce very few side-effects. Oro-pharyngeal candidiasis is the most troublesome although it occurs in only 5% of patients[10]. There is some evidence that candidiasis is related more to the frequency of inhalations than to the total dose of drug[11] and this is an argument for using the more concentrated inhalers and a twice daily regimen. Candidiasis which happens repeatedly with an aerosol, even with gargling or mouth rinsing after use, need not necessarily lead to discontinuation of the inhaled steroid. Changing to a powder inhaler, and particularly to a large-volume spacer device will usually allow the inhaled steroid to be continued. This is another aspect of the way in which greater familiarity with the range of inhalational devices available will enable general practitioners to manage their patients' asthma more effectively.

Reducing Morbidity: The Nebulizer Boom

Although nebulized bronchodilators are valuable in the management of acute asthma, at home and in hospital, their principal use is in the treatment of chronic asthma or chronic bronchitis and emphysema. Many patients, or their families, have heard of nebulizers and will ask their doctors about them. General practitioners may not feel they are in a position to refuse a patient a medical letter so that the patient can buy a machine, but if this is the case, a specialist should be asked to assess the patient. Patients have, in the past, obtained nebulizers in quite inappropriate circumstances[12] and general practitioners should recognize that a request for such a machine implies that the asthma is poorly controlled and should review all therapy. Much morbidity may be prevented by ensuring that patients are receiving drugs to suppress their asthma, such as inhaled steroids, rather than just given increased doses of bronchodilators. Curiously, doctors who are happy for their patients to have nebulizers are sometimes unhappy about what they see as excessive use of aerosols. It is possible that in the future doctors will feel under less pressure to provide nebulizers for their chronic asthmatics as it becomes more widely recognized that there is nothing magical about nebulized bronchodilators, and that the overwhelming reason for their success is the very large dose of drug inhaled. The pharmaceutical companies are already developing stronger versions of established β-agonist inhalers, mostly in powder form, as it seems probable that this form of therapy will obviate the need for nebulizers in some patients. In the meantime, those with chronic severe symptoms may be helped by being told that they should use their inhalers more liberally, and that it is not dangerous to do so provided that their other therapy is considered optimal. Nebulizers have become a fashion and asthma centres have become concerned, not only because of inappropriate use but also because of the enormous amount of time, effort and money which is involved in providing a nebulizer service, a service which can provide a backup when a patient's nebulizer breaks down, usually leading to subjective distress if not to objective deterioration in the asthma.

Reducing Morbidity: Patient Education

Asthma can be a chronic problem and, as for diabetes, the intention now is very much for patients to control their own disease whenever possible. As asthma is so common, it is simply not possible to see patients whenever a slight alteration in medication may be necessary and the aim must be to provide asthmatics with a basic understanding of their disease, their treatment and what to do if there is a problem. Teaching asthmatics about their disease is time-consuming because patients can only take in a small amount at a time, and every patient's capacity to understand is different. A small survey of adult asthmatics admitted to hospital or seen in our outpatient clinic recently showed that most patients had been told that bronchoconstriction was important in asthma, but other factors were much less commonly appreciated, and some, like airway inflammation, are important concepts in explaining

Table 5.1 Patients' understanding of asthma

72	*Frequency with which key words or phrases were mentioned* (%)
Bronchoconstriction	88
Inflammation of the airway	27
Excess mucus production	14
Allergy	9
Release of chemicals in the airway	0

how some treatments work (Table 5.1). Only 52% of patients said that they had been given an explanation of the nature of asthma, less than half of these by the general practitioner. Only 56% of patients took their medication as directed (the answers were being given to a final year pharmacy student and not to a doctor) and only the action of β-agonists was understood by most patients. Side-effects of drugs had not in general been discussed with patients, apart from the 26% who were aware of some of the long-term effects of steroids.

This dismal state of knowledge is not confined to asthma. The same small survey looked at two other chronic conditions, ischaemic heart disease and rheumatoid arthritis, and the same ignorance regarding pathology and the action of drugs was found. Patients with ischaemic heart disease complied with their drug taking more, possibly because they felt that failure to do so might be more life-threatening. The message is that doctors are not in general very good at explaining to patients what is wrong with them and why they should take certain forms of treatment to put things right. Nowadays, patients cannot be expected to comply with treatment unless they perceive a need for it and the days of taking medicine 'because the doctor tells you' are fast disappearing.

Several approaches to patient education are possible, and all may be needed in parallel. Verbal explanation is obviously the starting point, but few patients can retain much of what is said to them at one sitting. Written information is very helpful and many excellent leaflets are available, for example from the Asthma Society. These are of necessity general, and patients are more likely to retain something written personally for them, usually in the form of what each inhaler is for and what to do if the asthma gets worse[13]. The very basic minimum must be that all patients understand the difference between bronchodilators (relievers) and asthma-suppressing inhalers (preventers). Writing something down in longhand for the patient is quite time-consuming, and each doctor will have to work out the educational method which suits his practice best. It may be better to make several short appointments rather than one long one and to involve the practice nurses. Video material is likely to be used more in the future, and it should be possible for general practitioners to arrange for small groups of patients, particularly children, to look at such material together, perhaps with a nurse. The nurse can also make sure that patients are using their inhalers correctly. It is worth stressing that anyone who is responsible for teaching inhaler technique must be competent themselves. Many doctors and nurses are initially quite clueless with pressurized aerosols and fumble helplessly with powder inhalers.

Reduction in Mortality: Assessment and Treatment During Remissions

One of the most important questions to be answered over the next few years is whether asthma deaths can be reduced by applying the lessons learned from previous surveys. Most of the asthmatics who die have chronic severe asthma which has deteriorated over several days or weeks before death. Death is from hypoxia, due to a mixture of mucus plugging, oedema of the smaller airways and bronchoconstriction. The measurement of airflow obstruction by peak flow estimation is an indirect guide to asthma severity, and it should be our aim to

- Much of the present morbidity of asthma could be reduced by applying knowledge that we already have, and by using drugs already available. The first step is to consider the diagnosis of asthma more frequently, especially in children and in older patients who may be thought to have chronic bronchitis. Non-compliance with treatment is common, and may reflect poor understanding of the pathology of asthma by patients and poor education about medication. There is great scope for improving patients' knowledge and ability to manage their own treatment.

keep airflow obstruction to a minimum, within the limits imposed by the side-effects of available medication.

Many younger patients who die from asthma have fairly short-lasting attacks outside hospital, and sometimes there is a history which suggests that a marked degree of bronchial hyper-reactivity has been present for some time. The inference is that the final attack was due to sudden overwhelming bronchoconstriction due to an extreme reaction to a relatively mild asthma provocation. A graphic example was provided recently by a 32-year-old man who had previously been treated with salbutamol alone for his asthma. His resting lung function was normal, but he had given a story of 'going blue' and having trouble breathing after playing football sometimes. After one particular game he began to have difficulty in breathing and left the field to go to his car for his inhaler. He collapsed over the steering wheel, was quickly resuscitated and rushed to hospital where his asthma was easily controlled. Several months later he is mentally alert, but blind and unable to feed himself. This patient did not die from his respiratory arrest, but could well have done. He had an extreme degree of exercise-induced asthma, which is an everyday manifestation of bronchial hyper-reactivity. Other studies have shown that patients who have near-fatal attacks tend to have marked bronchial hyper-reactivity when they have recovered[14]. If patients with severe bronchial hyper-reactivity can be identified, it should be possible to reduce the hyper-reactivity by using drugs which suppress airway inflammation[15] and it should be practice to warn patients of their increased chances of severe asthma attacks so that they can have a plan of what to do in an emergency (see below).

Remission assessment of asthmatics is one means whereby mortality may be reduced by identifying patients at risk. Measurement of bronchial hyper-reactivity, though simple, is a technique for the hospital laboratory. A much easier technique is to measure peak flow rates over a period of days to assess the degree of diurnal variation, or morning dipping. A marked variation in peak flow over 24 hours indicates unstable asthma, and patients with this pattern regularly are at special risk (Figure 5.1). In the future, many more asthmatics should be assessed, if not regularly then at sometime when their asthma is considered to be stable by peak flow measurements at home.

Many specialists in Britain believe that the early use of drugs which suppress inflammation in the airways should be encouraged (e.g. inhaled steroids, sodium cromoglycate, nedocromil) because the airways inflammation is what leads to bronchial hyper-reactivity, the hallmark of asthma, and one of the causes of asthma deaths. Failure to use these drugs, with reliance on symptomatic bronchodilators only, is believed by some to be dangerous and to provide the potential for another increase in asthma deaths.

Reducing Mortality: Assessment and Treatment in Acute Episode

Analysis of the events surrounding asthma deaths outside hospital is a difficult and delicate task, involving doctors who may feel guilty or threatened and relatives who may feel bitter as well as distressed. As has been described in Chapter 2, the studies which have been carried out have uniformly shown that poor assessment of the attack by both doctor and patient, and inappropriate treatment characterized the management of most episodes which end in death[16]. Whether better management, including greater use of corticosteroids, will save lives remains to be seen, but this must surely be a hope for the future.

Patients who are considered to be particularly liable to severe asthma attacks should be provided with a plan of what to do. The rate of deterioration in asthma varies enormously, and fortunately most attacks come on over hours or days rather than minutes[17], so that there is time for appropriate action to be taken provided that the patient knows the problem. A supply of prednisolone tablets kept at home by the patient is essential, a nebulizer unit can be helpful in brittle asthmatics, and more rapid emergency self-help measures should be available to the few patients with a history of very sudden severe attacks. The suggested approach is summarized in Fig. 5.3.

The value of self-referral to hospitals is often debated. Self-referral to a specialist unit certainly provides the asthmatic with continuity of care, and often with more rapid access to treatment. Local factors clearly dictate the best policy. Large cities with many hospitals and frequent use of deputizing services by general practitioners are likely to find a self-referral system, such as the one pioneered in Edinburgh[18] particularly valuable. Smaller towns will probably find a less pressing need for a formal system, involving designated patients of which hospital wards, switchboards and the ambulance service have lists, but an informal system so that designated patients can

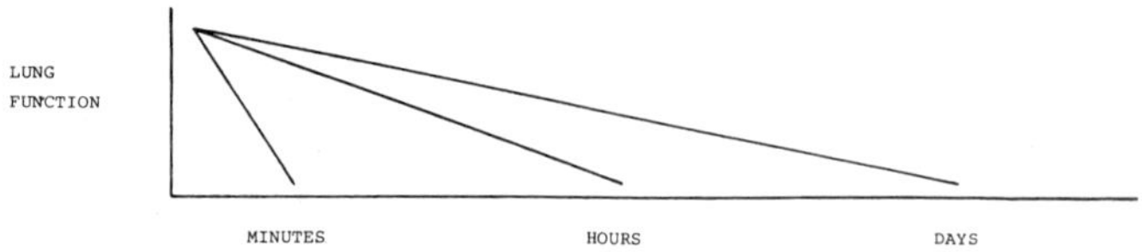

SYMPTOMS	Sudden onset of tightness and breathlessness	Gradual increase in tightness and breathlessness PFR ↓↓	Waking at night. Tightness lasting longer each morning PFR ↓
ACTION	S.C. or I.M. β agonist. Intranasal fenoterol Nebulizer if time 999 call.	Use more bronchodilator Check PFR If no better, prednisolone Call doctor/hospital ? self-referral	Increase bronchodilators and inhaled steroid. If no better, prednisolone Call doctor/hospital ? self-referral

Figure 5.3 Acute severe asthma and its management by the patient. Patients with very sudden severe attacks need to carry an emergency kit which may include an injectable *β*-agonist. A fenoterol inhaler with a nasal adaptor may be useful, as the drug may be rapidly absorbed from the nasal mucosa

telephone the hospital ward directly when in trouble can be extremely useful.

The aim of all such measures is to start effective treatment as soon as possible. Many general practitioners now have nebulizer units with which they can begin treatment, and of course some patients will have their own nebulizers. At present however, most patients with acute episodes do not receive nebulized bronchodilators unless they are admitted to hospital. Hospital admission, whether arranged by a general practitioner or because of an emergency ambulance call, involves an ambulance journey for most patients unless they are small children, and nebulized bronchodilators with oxygen can be very easily and safely administered by trained ambulance personnel[19]. This approach is likely to be used more widely in the future.

It should be emphasized that the management outlined above would be considered optimal in Britain at present. This is based on studies which have already been carried out, but asthma specialists would hope for a much greater application of this approach by general practitioners in the future. It has not been shown that better management will reduce overall asthma mortality, although it is possible to find anecdotal experiences from patients whose lives have been saved by appropriately timed treatment. Until general practitioners and their patients recognize the warning signs, and apply currently recommended measures, we shall never know how many asthma deaths are truly preventable.

- All studies have shown that many asthma deaths are preventable, in the sense that the treatment given before death was less than optimal by currently recommended standards. One of the great hopes for the future is that asthma mortality will fall as education of patients and doctors spreads.
- The severity of a patient's asthma should be assessed during remission and those considered at risk of severe acute attacks should be given a plan of what to do should their asthma deteriorate.

THE FUTURE: NEW DEVELOPMENTS

Epidemiology and Natural History

The prevalence of asthma and asthma mortality appear to vary a great deal between different countries, and this is an interesting field where further research in the future should prove rewarding. Table 5.2 shows the reported prevalence and mortality figures for several countries, and, in general, the mortality from asthma increases in proportion to the prevalence. The exception is in Sweden, where it is believed that local differences in death certification may be responsible for the higher apparent mortality. New Zealand has the highest prevalence of asthma in the world, outside local small communities such as Tristan da Cunha; this may be due to genetic factors in the Polynesian and Maori populations. Further work should clarify this. Asthma is hard to define, and at present, little information is available on prevalence in adult populations using standard criteria. Using such criteria surveys should then be able to separate real differences, which can be investigated, from differences which are simply due to diagnostic labelling. Real differences in prevalence can be looked at in terms of several factors, each of which can be examined, and differences in mortality can then be analysed to see whether mortality simply follows prevalence, or whether differences in severity or in the patterns of medical care may be partly responsible (Table 5.3).

Table 5.2 Asthma prevalence and mortality in different countries

	Prevalence (% population)	*Mortality* (deaths/100 000)
USA	3.2	1.4
UK	3.5	3.2
Sweden	2.5	6.5
Australia	8.5	4.0
New Zealand	12.2	8.0

Table 5.3 Possible factors affecting asthma prevalence and mortality in different countries[a]

Prevalence	*Mortality*
(Diagnostic labelling)	(Diagnostic labelling)
Genetic factors	Prevalence
Climate	Severity of asthma
Allergens	Patterns of care
Diet	Drugs
Infections/parasites	

[a] International comparisons are difficult without more uniform diagnosis and death certification.

There has certainly been an increased interest in the epidemiology of asthma over the past few years. International comparisons will help in the future and will be made possible only by standardizing coding practices. One possible reason for regional variations in asthma mortality is that the severity of asthma may vary; this can be examined by measuring bronchial hyper-reactivity using histamine or methacholine inhalation challenge in different populations. Some interesting results suggest that there may indeed be regions where bronchial hyper-reactivity is more prevalent[20] and it will be interesting to see whether there are areas where the severity of asthma, judged by bronchial hyper-reactivity, is more severe. There is some evidence which suggests that the prevalence of asthma and its severity (judged by the number of hospital admissions) may be increasing in Britain[21] and in other countries. How much of this is due to a heightened awareness among the public and general practitioners will need to be clarified.

Interesting differences exist in the drug treatment of asthma between countries[22]. In most of Europe the principal drugs used are the same, mainly inhaled β-agonists, inhaled steroids, oral theophylline and inhaled sodium cromoglycate, but the order in which they are used in chronic asthma varies. In Britain and Scandinavia, inhaled β-agonists and inhaled steroids are the drugs most widely used by specialists for maintenance treatment, whereas in France, Belgium, Austria and Germany, theophylline is the first-line maintenance treatment as it is in the USA. Theophylline is relatively unpopular among British specialists to the same degree that inhaled steroids are unpopular in France.

The value of other forms of treatment is also held to be quite different by specialists in different countries. Desensitization for allergic asthma is very rarely recommended in Britain and Northern Europe, while in France, Germany, Austria and Portugal, it is still quite commonly used. There is a mood of scepticism about it in the USA among chest physicians, although allergists of course still frequently recommend it.

It would be extremely interesting to compare asthma morbidity and mortality between countries which use different treatments for chronic asthma, and information which should be available within the next few years may well help to answer the question as to whether there is truly a proper way to treat asthma. In Britain, we tend to assume that the approach to treatment outlined in several chapters of this publication is the best, most rational and safest because Britain, like Scandinavia, has been in the forefront of drug development and evaluation. It would be gratifying to find this opinion born out by international comparison of different management strategies, and provide serious food for thought were there to be no differences in our favour.

The Cause of Asthma

What is understood of the pathogenesis of asthma has been discussed in Chapter 3. It will be apparent that bronchial inflammation and bronchial hyper-reactivity are important concepts, and considered central to asthma, but the factors which lead one particular individual to develop asthma are not understood. Genetic factors are important because asthma does tend to run in families as does the atopic tendency. Atopy does increase the chance of asthma occurring, but clearly additional factors are required other than just the ready tendency to demonstrate IgE-mediated responses, as shown by the 30% of the normal population who have positive skin tests. Many adults date the onset of their asthma to an acute respiratory infection, and in others the diagnosis begins following exposure to something at work.

It is not yet known whether the inflammation always precedes hyper-reactivity and asthma, or whether sometimes hyper-reactivity may be present first, so that an inflammatory stimulus may lead to asthma instead of mild bronchitis. The former seems more probable – inflammation preceding hyper-reactivity – and one piece of evidence for this is the variation in hyper-reactivity which occurs in asthmatics who are allergic to grass pollen, but who may have normal reactivity outside the pollen season[23]. The presence of chronic inflammation in the airways from many causes such as bronchiectasis and cystic fibrosis, may lead to altered reactivity and sometimes superimposed asthma. Usually, however, a chronic inflammatory response is characterized by a different type of cellular infiltrate from that which occurs in asthma and the reasons for this difference remain to be elucidated. Acute inflammation can also be caused by a variety of agents including infections and chemicals such as ozone. Transient hyper-reactivity can follow such inflammation in normal subjects[24]. One of the questions for the future is what causes inflammation of a particular type to persist in asthma, often after the initiating stimulus has gone.

In allergic asthma, mast cells sensitized with IgE are presumed to play an important role, and the mediators released from mast cells have been shown to have powerful effects on smooth muscle, on blood vessels and bronchial glands, as well as attracting secondary effector cells such as neutrophils. In allergic asthmatics symptoms may initially be related to acute allergen exposure, which seems straightforward but such individuals may present many years later with severe chronic asthma, and we do not know why their problem has persisted. It is possible that chronic mucosal damage may create a vicious circle where impaired mucociliary clearance and the presence of a damaged epithelium may allow inflammatory stimuli greater access to parts they normally would not reach.

Much of the asthma seen in older patients is non-atopic and assumed to be intrinsic rather than extrinsic. The same type of inflammatory response and the same hyper-reactivity are seen in these patients. Older patients often have asthma which is more persistent than younger asthmatics and, again, the factors involved are unknown. Some older patients (about 5%) are sensitive to aspirin and, as aspirin inhibits metabolism of arachidonic acid by cyclo-oxygenase, possibly leaving a larger substrate of arachidonic acid to be metabolized by the alternative 5-lipoxygenase pathway to leukotrienes, this at least suggests a specific area where there is an abnormality in some patients. Other older asthmatics become sensitized to substances they encounter at work, but often with a strange form of allergy which cannot be measured in terms of allergic antibody. The factors which predispose someone to develop occupational asthma are not understood, but it is usually unrelated to atopy. Several studies are being undertaken which will follow workers in specific occupations over several years to see whether any identifiable risk factors, for example pre-employment level of bronchial hyper-reactivity, can be found. Prospective studies like these are likely to be helpful in the future.

As implied above, we do not know why normal mechanisms do not cut short inflammation in asthmatics. It is not known why some children will grow out of their asthma, nor why some older asthmatics will continue to have asthma when removed from an occupational allergen. A recent study has re-emphasized this aspect of occupational asthma with respect to isocyanate exposure[25]. Isocyanates are widely used in the manufacture of polyurethanes, and it is estimated that up to 5% of exposed workers may develop asthma, usually after a relatively short time. This suggests that predisposing factors are important. Of 50 cases followed up, 82% continued to have some symptoms of asthma at least four years after cessation of exposure, and in only two cases was there a history of previous asthma in childhood. The authors commented that the continuing asthma of these patients was no different from asthma without an obvious initiating cause. It seems reasonable to hope that further insight into the factors controlling airway inflammation will be gained from studying such patients.

In the laboratory there have been enormous advances over the past few years, so that the cells involved (mast cells, eosinophils, basophils, neutrophils, lymphocytes, macrophages and platelets) can be harvested and examined separately. The chemicals which they produce can be measured, not just in the blood or in tissue preparations but in the airway and removed by bronchial lavage from asthmatic patients. The technical difficulties are enormous and there is much dispute between research groups as to the significance of different mediators and cells. Undoubtedly the future will see further advances and establish areas of agreement upon which further studies can be based. There is still room for more study of the pathology of asthma, in patients who have had the disease and in active asthmatics requiring lung resection for another reason, or dying of an unrelated cause. It will be particularly interesting to study the pathology in lungs from patients who once had asthma but have ceased to have it, or those who go on to develop asthma later – prospective and retrospective studies. One can imagine that such cases are not easy to find, but must slowly be accumulated from many centres.

There is a great deal to learn about the basic differences in cellular function and mediator release which distinguish asthmatic from normal airways. Once asthma is present, however, a number of different stimuli may act as triggers for attacks. Allergen inhalation is a clear example where an acute challenge produces effects due to the release of mediator substances from mast cells, but how the allergen reaches the target cells is not yet fully understood, nor is the role of the various primary and secondary mediators involved. Nocturnal asthma is a common event, occurring in most asthmatics when their asthma is slightly out of control, as one sign of increased bronchial hyper-reactivity. Its cause is still uncertain, although a great deal of research has been carried out[26]. As with so much in asthma a multifactorial pathogenesis is suspected, but no doubt the future will see a greater understanding of this distressing symptom.

Exercise-induced asthma is another manifestation of increased bronchial hyper-reactivity. Over the past 20 years an enormous literature has developed, and gradually the measure of agreement between investigators has increased. The feature of exercise now generally believed to be important is the associated hyperventilation of relatively dry and cool air (unconditioned by the nose). This appears to cause a mucosal effect leading both to the release of mediator substances and to the stimulation of nerve endings[27], the relative amounts of each differing between individuals (and perhaps within one individual at different times, although this has not been shown). It appears at present to be the dryness of the air, causing evaporation of water from the mucosa to humidify the air, which is most important, and current work is attempting to assess whether it is the subsequent change in osmolarity which somehow acts as a trigger for asthma. The future will certainly see further advances in our understanding of exercise-induced asthma and in turn may help us to understand more of the asthma disease process in general.

New Treatments

Future advances in the treatment of asthma range from relatively minor improvements in drug formulation and delivery to the development of completely new drugs with new modes of action. Table 5.4 shows some of the more imminent future new treatments.

The dry powder inhaler has been of great benefit to the many patients who cannot use pressurized aerosols correctly. One of its disadvantages is that it is slightly inconvenient to use and has to be reloaded with a new capsule each time. Multidose powder inhalers are likely to be available soon which can carry at least a day's supply of capsules and which will reload automatically. Other pharmaceutical companies are likely to move into the dry powder field, so that, for example, anticholinergic drugs as well as β-agonist drugs and corticosteroids can be given in this way. A further future trend in dry powder inhalers will be the development of high-dose β-agonist capsules. This has already been mentioned in discussing the use of nebulizers. Large doses of β-agonist drugs have a larger immediate effect but they also cause a more sustained bronchodilatation. This may be onc way of reducing the frequency of inhalations, where a continued effect is

Table 5.4 Future developments in asthma treatment

Drug delivery	High dose powder capsules Multidose powder inhalers Powder versions of more drugs
Bronchodilators	Longer-acting β agonists Beta-agonist pro-drugs Enprofylline
Steroids	Longer-acting inhaled steroids Greater local/systemic effect
Non-steroid anti-inflammatory	Nedocromil
Mediator antagonists	Anti-leukotriene C_4, D_4, E_4 Anti-prostaglandin D_2 Anti-thromboxane Others
Diet	Additional fatty acids Less food additives
Immunotherapy	Better vaccines
Other	Yoga, acupuncture

required, and thus improve patient compliance. Trials are at present in progress to assess this approach.

New Bronchodilators

The pharmaceutical companies with a major interest in asthma are continually seeking to improve their products. In the area of β-adrenergic agonists the available drugs are already excellent, but have a relatively short duration of action of approximately four hours following a standard dose. Drugs have been developed with a longer duration of action and are currently undergoing clinical trials. Provided that the rapid onset of action is not sacrificed this should be a useful advance and improve asthma during the day, when patients often forget their inhalers, and at night when patients might have symptoms in the early hours of the morning. Another occasional problem with β-agonists is the occurrence of minor side-effects such as tremor and palpitations. These are largely obviated by the use of inhalers rather than tablets, but nevertheless occur from time to time. Pro-drugs have been developed which, taken orally, are selectively converted into active drug only in the bronchi. It is hoped that these compounds may allow twice daily dosing, while providing great specificity for the airways. Whether side-effects will be less than with inhaled drugs remains to be seen.

The use of theophylline as a bronchodilator has already been discussed and concern expressed over its rather high incidence of side-effects when used in doses which cause reasonable bronchodilatation. Many xanthine derivatives have been examined to see whether it is possible to separate the effects of bronchodilatation from the most dangerous side-effects, and it appears that this can be achieved. Many xanthines are bronchodilators, but one particular compound (enprofylline) (Fig. 5.4) has been extensively studied because of its apparent freedom from many of the extrapulmonary

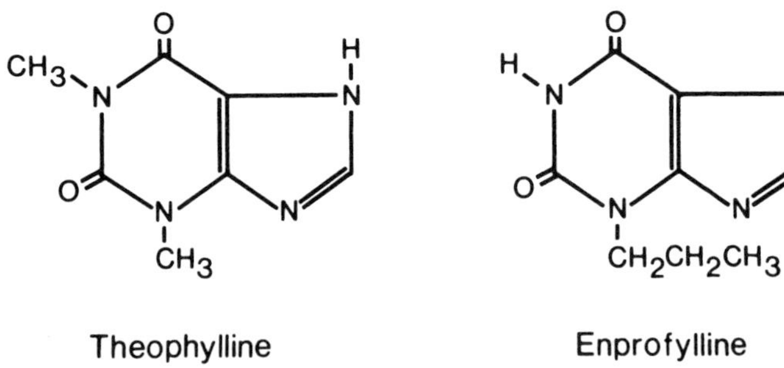

Figure 5.4 Structures of theophylline and enprofylline. Theophylline is an adenosine antagonist while enprofylline is not. Both are bronchodilators

effects of theophylline. The mode of action of theophylline is still unknown. Traditional teaching is that theophylline prevents the breakdown of cyclic AMP by inhibiting phosphodiesterase in cells but, while this may happen *in vitro*, the concentration of drug achievable *in vivo* is probably much too small for phosphodiesterase inhibition to be significant. Theophylline is a powerful antagonist of adenosine, which is produced in many tissues of the body by cells under stress and perhaps acts as a distress signal. It is believed that adenosine antagonism may be responsible for many of the undesirable effects of theophylline such as convulsions, anxiety, restlessness and increased gastric acid secretion. Enprofylline lacks appreciable adenosine antagonist effect[28] and may therefore prove to be better tolerated and safer. Unfortunately, it may still cause some centrally-mediated nausea. Since enprofylline appears to be at least as effective a bronchodilator as theophylline, adenosine antagonism does not explain theophylline's mechanism of bronchodilatation, and this remains poorly understood. One further possible benefit of enprofylline is that it is metabolized in a different way from theophylline and excreted largely unchanged by the kidneys. This reduces the potential for drug interactions. Enprofylline is just beginning large-scale clinical trials and its role in asthma therapy will be known in the next few years.

New corticosteroids

Corticosteroids remain the most valuable drugs for treating all but mild asthma. Orally, their effects are well known and it is unlikely that new advances will be made in this field relevant to asthma. Steroids with more powerful glucocorticoid (anti-inflammatory) effects may be produced, but the side-effects from chronic administration will be increased in parallel. Prednisolone remains, and is likely to continue to be, the oral steroid of choice[29]. The revolution in steroid therapy in asthma came with the development of steroids which produced powerful local effects when inhaled, without significant systemic absorption. New inhaled steroids are being produced which will accentuate the local surface anti-inflammatory effect, while minimizing systemic activity and adrenal suppression even at high doses. This is usually achieved by ensuring that a compound is rapidly broken down to an inactive metabolite if it enters the circulation. There is also potential for a longer-lasting topical effect as current drugs must be given twice daily to maintain control of asthma.

New Mast Cell Stabilizing Drugs

It is doubtful whether any drug currently used exerts its main anti-asthma effect through mast cell stabilization. Sodium cromoglycate and ketotifen both have *in vitro* effects of this kind, but so do many drugs which are quite ineffective in asthma. Sodium cromoglycate has been promoted for many years as a mast cell stabilizing agent, but there is much evidence that it does not work in this way[30] and its true mode of action, like that of theophylline, is unclear. Ketotifen is a weak drug in asthma but a powerful antihistamine, and although quite widely-used in Europe, British specialists have found it to be rather ineffective in clinical practice. Many companies have spent large sums of money on developing an oral mast cell stabilizing drug, but this approach has not produced clinically useful agents[30] and I do not believe that it will in the future. Part of this relates to the difficulty in devising *in vitro* tests which will predict *in vivo* effects, and part to the less central role which the mast cell is now believed to occupy in chronic asthma.

Anti-inflammatory drugs

There has been an important new development in this field which is likely to have an impact on the management of asthma in the future. Nedocromil sodium is a drug which has been under investigation for some years and is now available on prescription. The drug is delivered from a pressurized aerosol and recommended for use in adults rather than children (in whom little experience has been gained). It is relatively expensive. Nedocromil is in some ways related to sodium cromoglycate, but it has an anti-inflammatory activity[31] and has been shown to reduce the bronchial response to non-allergic forms of bronchial challenge such as inhalation of sulphur dioxide and cold air as well as exercise. It is not a steroid and possesses no bronchodilator activity. Nedocromil has been shown to be effective in long-term clinical trials, where it has been used either as a replacement for inhaled steroids, or for an oral steroid sparing effect[32]. The evidence so far suggests that this compound is less effective than inhaled steroids, but further studies will show whether it can produce improvement when the dose of inhaled steroids cannot be increased without significant systemic effect. It cannot yet be recommended as first line therapy until more experience is gained.

Enzyme inhibitors/activators

Many drugs which are already used in asthma exert their actions by affecting various enzymes. For example, β-agonists activate adenylate cyclase to produce cyclic AMP and steroids appear to work by inhibiting phospholipase A_2, the enzyme responsible for breaking down cell membrane phospholipids to arachidonic acid. As more is learned of the various mediators in asthma, and their mode of production, it will become possible to develop compounds which will interfere with the generation of harmful mediators or enhance the production of beneficial substances. An example is provided by the two pathways of arachidonic acid metabolism. Inhibitors of cyclo-oxygenase already exist in the form of aspirin-like drugs, but more asthmatics are made worse by aspirin than are made better. Inhibitors of the alternative lipoxygenase pathway, which produces leukotrienes, have been developed for trial and will certainly be investigated further in the future. A thromboxane synthetase inhibitor is also available but extensive studies have not yet been performed.

Mediator antagonists

Many substances have been identified as possible asthma mediators and it is possible to examine their roles by interfering with their release (mast cell stabilizing drugs), their synthesis (steroids), or antagonizing their actions on cells (antihistamines). Not only does this increase what is known about asthma but it gives the opportunity to develop drugs which may be effective treatments. So far, however, no single mediator has been found which is so important that antagonizing it results in clinical benefit. Antihistamines are a classical example. It is known that histamine is important in asthma, but though laboratory tests can show reduction of asthma in challenge situations when antihistamines are used[33], even the modern selective H_1-receptor antagonists are rather unhelpful in day-to-day asthma. This is presumably because of the large number of other cells and mediators which are also involved. Drugs which may be helpful are antagonists of leukotrienes, particularly LTC_4, LTD_4, and LTE_4 (which make up what was known as slow reacting substance of anaphylaxis, SRS-A) and of the particularly potent prostaglandin D_2. Thromboxane antagonists are already available. Much work will be done in the near future using these mediator antagonists, but it is hard to imagine how one single compound will prove useful in such a complicated pharmacological situation. There may be more scope for the clinical use of combinations of various antagonists.

Non-drug treatments

Future developments in the management of asthma may involve more than new drugs. There has for some time been interest in other approaches, some from conventional medicine and some more associated with alternative, or complementary, medicine. One approach which is being explored is that of modification of the diet. This has two aspects, the first of which is to increase the proportion of certain fatty acids in the diet, and the second is to remove from the diet potentially harmful substances. The theoretical basis of increasing the dietary

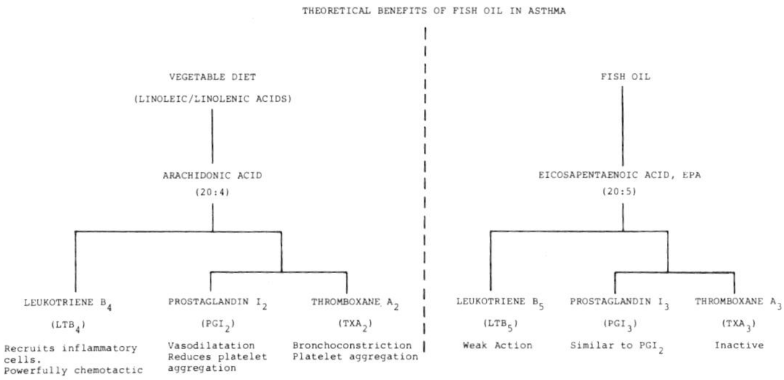

Figure 5.5 The theory behind fish oil supplementation. In cardiovascular disease, the benefits are related to reduction in TXA_2 activity when replaced with TXA_3. In asthma, the weaker chemotactic effect of LTB_5 compared to LTB_4 may also be beneficial. This has not yet been shown in practice

amount of certain fatty acids is shown in Fig. 5.5. A normal diet provides large amounts of linoleic and linolenic acids for cell membranes and these form arachidonic acid (also known as eicosapentaenoic acid) which has a chain of 20 carbon atoms but 4 double bonds (hence 20:4). Fish oil contains large amounts of eicosapentaenoic acid, which also has a chain of 20 carbon atoms but 5 double bonds (hence 20:5). This can act as an alternative substrate for the lipoxygenase and cyclo-oxygenase pathways leading to leukotrienes, prostaglandins and thromboxanes, all with one more double bond than they would have if derived from arachidonic acid (hence LTB_5 instead of LTB_4). These compounds in some cases have much weaker actions than the usual metabolites, and may therefore cause less inflammation and be less powerfully chemotactic. It has been shown that dietary enrichment with these fish oil fatty acids can cause significant changes along these lines in human neutrophils and monocytes when examined *in vitro*[34]. Preliminary studies in asthmatics are being undertaken, although the earliest results suggest that any clinical effect is likely to be small. Taking extra fish oil is not for everyone's palate and the diet provides a significant extra calorie load.

Many asthmatics believe that their condition is caused by extrinsic factors and if these are not inhaled then they must be present in the diet. Few would disagree that allergy to certain foods and to food additives can be a problem for some individuals[35]. At present, an elimination diet is the only way to prove this, a process which can be tedious and expensive. It is not something to be recommended for all late-onset asthmatics, but much will be learned of the effect of modern dietary constituents on asthma over the next few years. It is a field in which a great deal of pseudo-science exists, and asthmatics who seek help in some private allergy clinics should be told to read the *Which* report on food allergy[36] which found considerable discrepancies in the advice which several genuine sufferers were given in different clinics.

Treatment of asthma itself has been given by several complementary therapies, including hypnosis, acupuncture and yoga[37,38,39]. Objective evaluation of the effect on asthma is difficult but the results have been favourable in some individuals. This contrasts with the considerable and more reliable beneficial effect of current drug treatment, but there is no reason to dissuade patients from undertaking these therapies provided they do not suddenly discontinue all their standard medication. No doubt more will be known about the value of techniques such as meditation and acupuncture in particular in the future, and the best way to use these ancient disciplines in our own culture.

Immunotherapy (desensitization) occupies a place between conventional medicine and alternative medicine in many specialists' minds in Britain. It is still enormously popular in some European countries, but there is little evidence of benefit when it is used routinely in all asthmatics who show skin sensitivity to allergens. Desensitization can occasionally be useful in grass pollen or house dust mite sensitive patients but it should be remembered that it is potentially dangerous, even lethal[40], as well as being time-consuming and expensive. One of the reasons that allergen extracts are unsatisfactory at present is that they are relatively impure, and an extract may contain many different allergens. Improved quality and purity of these extracts in the future should enable more success to be achieved, but the other reason that desensitization fails is that single allergen exposure amenable to desensitization is very rarely the only cause of continuing troublesome asthma.

Patients' expectations

Many patients who are newly-diagnosed as having asthma have unrealistic expectations of a cure. Some will spend a lot of time and money in attending allergy clinics or alternative medical practitioners in the hope that they can be freed from the need to take drugs. Few will achieve this goal. It should be explained to patients that there is no cure, nor is there likely to be, but that certain extrinsic causes can be investigated. The list of these will obviously increase in the future and the number of truly intrinsic asthmatics perhaps diminish. Most patients will need to take drugs, and patients should be left in no doubt as to the efficacy of current medication (perhaps even greater efficacy in the future) and the freedom from side-effects which is greater than for any other long-term medication because of its inhaled locally-acting nature. Patients will expect, and should receive, a sympathetic explanation of the nature of asthma and its treatment, and the doctor should state what he is trying to achieve. The doctor should be flexible enough to tailor the exact treatment regimen to the patient's own personal circumstances and inclinations, while using drugs which he knows will be effective, and standing firm against unreasonable demands and prejudices.

- Future increase in our knowledge of asthma will require greater research into the causes of airway inflammation, what causes it to turn on and off, and what causes persistent inflammation in the absence of any obvious extrinsic factor.
- International comparisons of asthma prevalence and mortality will provide valuable information about the most effective drug regimens for treating asthma.
- New treatment for asthma will involve improvements to existing delivery systems and drugs, as well as entirely new compounds. The new compounds will include anti-inflammatory agents, as well as specific inhibitors and antagonists to the increasingly large number of putative asthma mediators.
- Whatever new forms of treatment become available, patients will expect to be told why the doctor recommends a particular regimen for them. A patient who is unhappy with the treatment is likely to be non-compliant but, conversely, there is nothing like effective treatment to make people feel happier with themselves and their doctor.

REFERENCES

1. Rees, J. (1984). ABC of asthma: Definition and diagnosis. *Br. Med. J.*, **288,** 1370–2
2. Connolly, C. K. (1987). Falsely high peak expiratory flow readings due to acceleration in the mouth. *Br. Med. J.*, **294,** 285
3. Hodson, M. E. (1986). Are there problems with the efficacy and safety of high dose inhaled steroids? *Res. Clin. Forums,* **8,** 39–43
4. Speight, A. N. P., Lee, D. A. and Hay, E. N. (1983). Underdiagnosis and undertreatment of asthma in childhood. *Br. Med. J.*, **286,** 1253–6
5. O'Byrne, P. M., Morris, M., Roberts, R. and Hargreave, F. E. (1982). Inhibition of the bronchial response to respiratory heat exchange by increasing doses of terbutaline sulphate. *Thorax,* **37,** 913–7
6. Henriksen, J. M. (1985). Effect of inhalation of corticosteroids on exercise-induced asthma: randomized double blind crossover study of budesonide in asthmatic children. *Br. Med. J.*, **291,** 248–9
7. Fitch, K. D., Morton, A. R. and Blanksby, B. A. (1976). Effects of swimming training on children with asthma. *Arch. Dis. Child.*, **51,** 190–4
8. Paterson, I. C. and Crompton, G. K. (1976). The use of pressurized aerosols by asthmatic patients. *Br. Med. J.*, **1,** 76–7
9. Hartley, J. P. R. (1986). Theophylline therapy. *Resp. Dis. Pract.*, **3,** 14–19
10. Milne, L. J. R. and Crompton, G. K. (1974). Beclomethasone dipropionate and oropharyngeal candidiasis. *Br. Med. J.*, **3,** 797–8
11. Smith, M. J. and Hodson, M. E. (1983). High-dose beclomethasone inhaler in the treatment of asthma. *Lancet,* **1,** 265–8
12. Laroche, C. M., Harries, A. V. K., Newton, R. C. F. and Britton, M. G. (1985). Domiciliary nebulisers in asthma: a district survey. *Br. Med. J.*, **290,** 1611–3
13. Burge, P. S. (1984). Getting the best out of bronchodilator therapy. In: Clark, T. J. H. (ed) *Bronchodilator Therapy,* pp. 58–75. (Auckland: Adis Press)
14. Woolcock, A. J. (1986). Worldwide differences in asthma prevalence and mortality. *Chest,* **90** (Suppl), 40S–5S
15. Hartley, J. P. R. (1986). The early use of inhaled steroids in adults. *Res. Clin. Forums,* **8,** 29–35
16. British Thoracic Society. (1982). Deaths from asthma in two regions of England. *Br. Med. J.*, **285,** 1251–6
17. Arnold, A. G., Lane, D. J. and Zapata, E. (1982). The speed of onset and severity of acute sevee asthma. *Br. J. Dis. Chest,* **76,** 157–63
18. Crompton, G. K. and Grant, I. W. B. (1975). Edinburgh emergency asthma admission service. *Br. Med. J.*, **4,** 680–2
19. Turton, C. W. G., Chamberlain, D. A. C., Miller, G. and Grainger, R. (1987). Can ambulance men give nebulised salbutamol? *Thorax,* **42,** 231–2
20. Burney, P., Britton, J., Chinn, S., Tattersfield, A., Platt, H., Papacosta,

A. O. and Kelson, M. (1986). The relationship between the bronchial response to inhaled histamine and 24 hour sodium excretion. *Thorax,* **41,** 240–1

21. Khot, A., Burn, R., Evans, N., Lenney, C. and Lenney, W. (1984). Seasonal variation and time trends in childhood asthma in England and Wales 1975–81. *Br. Med. J.,* **289,** 235–7
22. Vermeire, P. A., Wittesaele, W. M., Janssens, E. and De Backer, W. A. (1986). European audit of asthma therapy. *Chest,* **90** (Suppl), 58S–61S
23. Cockcroft, D. W., Berschied, B. A., Murdock, K. Y. and Gore, B. P. (1985). Sensitivity and specificity of histamine PC_{20} measurements in a random population. *J. Allergy Clin. Immunol.,* **75,** 151
24. Empey, D. W., Laitinen, L. A., Jacobs, L., Gold, W. and Nadel, J. A. (1976). Mechanisms of bronchial hyperreactivity in normal subjects after upper respiratory tract infection. *Am. Rev. Resp. Dis.,* **113,** 131–9
25. Lozewicz, S., Assoufi, B. K., Hawkins, R. and Newman Taylor, A. J. (1987). Outcome of asthma induced by isocyanates. *Br. J. Dis. Chest,* **81,** 14–22
26. Barnes, P. J. (1984). Nocturnal asthma: mechanisms and treatment. *Br. Med. J.,* **288,** 1397–8
27. Lee, T. H., Anderson, S. D. (1985). Heterogeneity of mechanisms in exercise induced asthma. *Thorax,* **40,** 481–7
28. Persson, C. G. A., Karlsson, J-A. and Erjefalt, I. (1982). Differentiation between bronchodilation and universal adenosine antagonism among xanthine derivatives. *Life Sci.,* **30,** 2181–9
29. Lewis, L. D. and Cochrane, G. M. (1986). Systemic steroids in chronic severe asthma. *Br. Med. J.,* **292,** 1289
30. Stokes, T. C. and Morley, J. (1981). Prospects for an oral Intal. *Br. J. Dis. Chest,* **75,** 1–14
31. Eady, R. P. (1986). The pharmacology of nedocromil sodium. *Eur. J. Resp. Dis.,* **69** (Suppl. 147), 112–19
32. Holgate, S. T. (1986). Clinical evaluation of nedocromil sodium in asthma. *Eur. J. Resp. Dis.,* **69** (Suppl. 147): 149–59
33. Holgate, S. T., Emanuel, M. B. and Howarth, P. H. (1985). Astemizole and other H_1-antihistamine drug treatment of asthma. *J. Allergy Clin. Immunol.,* **76,** 375–80
34. Lee, T. H., Hoover, R. L., Williams, J. D., Sperling, R. I., Ravalese, J., Spur, B. W., Robinson, D. R., Corey, E. J., Lewis, R. A. and Austen, K. F. (1985). Effect of dietary enrichment with eicosapentaenoic acid and docosahexaenoic acids on *in vitro* neutrophil and monocyte leukotriene generation and neutrophil function. *N. Engl. J. Med.,* **312,** 1217–24
35. Mygind, N. (1986). Gastro-intestinal reactions and food sensitivity. In: Mygind, N. (ed) *Essential Allergy,* pp. 137–59. (Oxford: Blackwell Scientific Publications)
36. Allergies to food. *Which?* Jan. (1987) 6–8
37. Ewer, T. C. and Stewart, D. E. (1986). Improvement in bronchial hyperresponsiveness in patients with moderate asthma after treatment with a hypnotic technique. *Br. Med. J.,* **293,** 1129–32

38. Chu, S. S. and Pearce, S. J. (1983). Acupuncture point stimulation in bronchial asthma. *Thorax,* **38,** 221–2
39. Nagarathna, R. and Nagendra, H. R. (1985). Yoga for bronchial asthma: a controlled study. *Br. Med. J.,* **291,** 1077–9
40. Desensitizing vaccines (allergen extracts) and anaphylaxis. Circular from Committee on Safety of Medicines, 8 Oct (1986)

6

CASE REPORTS

REPORT NUMBER 1

An 11-year-old girl was referred in August 1981.

GPs letter: 'Thank you for seeing this young girl who became wheezy when she was two years of age. Recently she has had increasingly frequent episodes which are more severe. She has no rhonchi in her chest today but an upper respiratory tract infection. She is allergic to ?horses, hay, bananas, nuts, cherries, house-dust, feathers, rabbit, etc. She is taking Piriton, Phenergan, Phyllocontin and Ventolin inhaler. Please would you advise about further management.'

Response: 'Many thanks indeed for your helpful letter and for asking me to see this young girl. Her brother has hay fever and eczema. Grandmother had asthma and mother has 'allergy' problems. Rachel has been asthmatic from birth but recently there is progressive breathlessness, wheeze, cough on exercise and at night. Examination was satisfactory. FEV_1 2.0 l, PEFR 250 l/min. Chest X-ray showed right upper lobe pneumonitis – probably allergic in aetiology. Skin tests showed strong reaction to grass pollen, silver birch, horse, cat and mixed nuts. There was no reaction to eggs or milk.

The diagnosis of extrinsic asthma is not in doubt. I think she would benefit from regular use of salbutamol rotacapsules.

Phyllocontin and Phenergan could be stopped and she could take Intal and Becotide twice a day. I will see her again shortly.'

Progress: On review in September 1981, she was well but said that Becotide she found to be unnecessary and required a small dose of Phenergan at night. In April 1982, in spite of regular treatment, her symptoms were much worse. She was given depo-medrone (IM) with immediate response. PEFR rising to 370 l/min and she stopped all medication except salbutamol before exercise. This 'line' of management continued, i.e. depo-medrone every three months till April 1986, then stopped. The girl remained active and well. However, in August 1986 her asthma and rhinitis recurred in a mild form and easily controlled using Becotide inhaler and Beconase nasal spray.

Comment: Extrinsic asthma in girls tends to be more of a problem than in boys, often progressing into adulthood with added factors of menstrual and hormonal influences.

REPORT NUMBER 2

A 9-year-old boy was referred in November 1982.

GPs letter: 'Thank you for seeing this young boy who has a long history of catarrh, irritating eyes and intermittent wheezing. On examination today he has large tonsils. His chest is clear of rhonchi.

Please would you advise about further investigation regarding allergies in this child. He has been given Piriton 2 mg bd by —— but this has not helped. He is now using Intal plain spincaps regularly and Phenergan 10 mg nocte.'

Response: This schoolboy's father has sinusitis but there is no other family history of relevance. For a number of years he has had recurring rhinitis and conjunctivitis and now has exercise-induced asthma. On examination there was some tenderness on palpation of his sinuses, his tonsils were rather large and inflamed. His chest was clear.

FEV_1 was 1.5 l, FVC 1.85 l and PEFR 270 l/min. Chest X-ray was normal.

This is the syndrome of rhinitis/conjunctivitis/asthma. Skin test results may be interesting. I have asked him to continue with the Intal inhaler two or three times a day and Phenergan at night.'

Progress: Allergy tests (prick):
House dust mites 20 mm
Cultured rye 12 mm
Grass pollen 12 mm
House dust 10 mm
Aspergillus, yeast, rabbit, feathers, cat, dog – negative.

Symptoms not under control, advised to take Becotide twice a day alongside salbutamol and Intal used for the next six weeks. On review – no improvement. Mother rearranged bedroom, etc. to minimize problems from house dust mite. Not keen on a programme of desensitization. Therefore depo-medrone 40 mg given in February 1983. This caused dramatic improvement. Phenergan, Intal and salbutamol stopped. Becotide used rarely before exercise. Depo-medrone repeated every three to four months for a year. Then stopped and asked to recommence Intal, salbutamol and Becotide regularly. Soon the child became, in mother's words, 'miserable, coughing, wheezing and sneezing'. Depo-medrone recommenced with prompt improvement – treatment continued till July 1986. The boy now 13 years of age feeling very well. Depo-medrone stopped, salbutamol and Becotide continued and advised to use it when necessary. On review in October 1986 and May 1987 remains well (PEFR 350 l/min; weight gain 24.1 kg (1982) to 49.1 kg (1987).

Comment: This story demonstrates that extrinsic asthma, common in boys of this age, can be difficult to control with inhaled medication alone. The child 'suffers' at school and often fails to thrive. Injections of a depo-steroid given intermittently may be indicated in these children and provided they are kept under close review, should be regarded as safe.

REPORT NUMBER 3

A Kenyan-born, 29-year-old lady was referred in December 1984.

GPs letter: 'Thank you very much for seeing this chronic asthmatic who is 26 weeks pregnant. She had a bad flare-up in the middle of November, when my partner, Dr —— had to give her intravenous hydrocortisone and a course of prednisone. She is again very wheezy and breathless this morning, and I have started her on Ventolin rotahaler with 400 μg capsules. As she is pregnant, we are rather limited in the choice of bronchodilators, and I felt that she should have specialist cover while she is pregnant. I should be most grateful for your advice on management.'

Response: 'Many thanks indeed for asking me to see this accountant who is a non-smoker and has had childhood asthma. Her father was also asthmatic. It looks as if in the last 11 weeks of her pregnancy she has had two episodes of severe asthma, both of these needing intravenous hydrocortisone and short courses of prednisone. It is interesting to note that during one of her attacks her PEFR was only 120 l/min. Today it was 340.

She admits to allergy to house dust and 'the mite'. We may in future consider a programme of densitization. I have reassured her about any possible harmful effects to the foetus from the recent course of prednisone and have told her that it is much more important to control the asthma at this late stage. I have asked her to take salbutamol inhaler on regular basis, to acquire a peak flow meter and achieve a PEFR >300 l/min. I have also prescribed Tymasil which she may find useful against the house dust mite. I will see her again shortly.'

Progress: Six weeks later, on review, admitted to have taken a course of prednisone and on regular salbutamol had PEFR >320 l/min. Had three further weeks of pregnancy to continue treatment. Delivered a normal baby in March 1985.

In December 1985, her first attendance at the clinic since delivery, she admitted to progressive deterioration in her asthma, with continual cough and wheeze. She had taken salbutamol, Intal, Becotide and oral prednisone (5–15 mg daily) and yet PEFR was rarely above 140 l/min. Chest X-ray showed 'sputum plugs'. On prednisone for six months she had gained 10 kg in weight and was not prepared to continue any longer.

Patient was supplied with home nebulizer with recommendation to use salbutamol three or four times a day followed by inhaled Becotide and use minimum dose of prednisone. This produced *no* symptomatic improvement and PEFR remained below 160 l/min.

She was then given triamcinolone (Kenalog) 80 mg im. This resulted in rapid improvement. She felt that other medication was not necessary and kept her PEFR >340 l/min.

She remained well till June 1986 when asthma had recurred (PEFR <110 l/min). She declined to take prednisone, Becotide or Intal which she felt had not been of much benefit. Allergy tests (prick) again confirmed very significant allergic response to house dust and house dust mite. A further injection of triamcinolone was given and asked to try ipratropium bromide (Atrovent) inhaler regularly and obtain IGR-S spray against the house dust mite. There was immediate improvement which has been maintained. There has been no further need of triamcinolone and she has taken Atrovent and salbutamol regularly. PEFR varies between 270–340 l/min.

Comment: This patient demonstrates very clearly:

(1) some asthmatics are difficult to manage;

(2) unpredictable nature of the condition; and

(3) triamcinolone succeeded where other treatment not so effective.

REPORT NUMBER 4

A 67-year-old retired British Gas employee was referred in November 1982.

GPs letter: 'Thank you for seeing this man who has very troublesome asthma. He has had it for years but it has bothered him more during the past two years. He has been under Dr —— at —— before his move here. In 1981 he had a respiratory arrest in ——. Following his attendance there with severe asthma he has been on oral steroids for most of the past 10 years. He has not worked for some time because of incapacity due to his chest.

He is on heroic therapy at present and is still wheezy despite prednisolone averaging 15 mg daily, Phyllocontin one bd, aminophylline suppositories one nocte, bromhexine four daily, Ventolin inhaler too frequently, and Ventolin spandets one nocte. I have again encouraged him to restart and regularly use his Becotide inhaler and to increase Ventolin spandets to two a day. He has required iv/im bronchodilators on three occasions in the last month.

I wonder if you feel he would benefit from using a Ventolin nebulizer at home and would value your advice'.

Response: 'Many thanks for your helpful letter and for asking me to see this patient who is an ex-smoker (6 years). There is strong family history of neoplastic disease.

He has had what he calls a 'recurrent sinusitis' and removal of nasal polyps. Over the past 14 years there has been progressive breathlessness, with wheezing, sputum, cough and nocturnal distress. He has been on prednisolone over the whole length of this illness.

On examination he has hyperinflated chest. Forced expiratory time was prolonged. There was widespread polyphonic wheeze. FEV_1 1.5 l, FVC 2.85 l, and PFR 310 l/min. Chest X-ray showed low flat hemidiaphragm and left basal inflammatory change.

He therefore has steroid-dependent severe intrinsic asthma

with nasal polyps. It would be preferable to reduce oral prednisolone and improve his lung function. To this aim I am trying Triamcinolone (Kenalog) and have asked him to reduce the prednisolone to 2.5 mg daily taking Becotide inhaler twice daily and salbutamol as required. He will now use aminophylline suppositories only when necessary.'

Progress: When seen again six weeks later, he had been able to reduce prednisolone to 2.5 mg a day, decided to reduce Becotide to one puff twice a day and had used salbutamol occasionally. FEV_1, FVC and PEFR remained unchanged but symptomatically he felt better.

A further triamcinolone 80 mg im was given and advised to stop prednisolone altogether. This he was able to do. He received two further triamcinolone injections at six weekly intervals – the interval between injections changed to three months. Rib fractures developed in September 1983 due to alcohol-induced osteoporosis but on reducing alcohol, no further fractures have been noted.

In July 1985 he was admitted to hospital with acute exacerbation of asthma due to lobar pneumonia. He was given iv antibiotics, hydrocortisone and oral prednisolone and improved. Prednisolone was withdrawn in August 1985. He continued triamcinolone, now every few months when PEFR fell below 200 but took Becotide and salbutamol regularly.

When seen in March 1987 he was well, PEFR 280 l/min, emigrating to Spain. His wife, a nurse has undertaken to give triamcinolone when necessary.

Comment: This patient, an intrinsic asthmatic was able to stop prednisolone after 14 years needing only one course during hospital admission with acute severe asthma. His lifestyle has improved, he has lost 6 kg in weight (glucocorticosteroid effect) and drug therapy is relatively 'simple'. He has no evidence of proximal muscle weakness or bruising – two main side-effects of triamcinolone therapy. His PEFR, FEV, FVC have remained at 65% of predicted levels.

REPORT NUMBER 5

A 70-year-old retired aviation inspector was referred in February 1981.

GPs letter: 'Thank you for seeing this patient who appeared to develop asthma this summer at the age of 70 years.

He developed an intractable cough for which no obvious cause could be found (CXR normal) and did not respond to antibiotics, expectorants, etc. and Ventolin 2 mg one bd made him feel unwell.

When I saw him first mid-October I found his BP 200/110, P 80 and concluding he had asthma I started him on Intal plain tds and Phyllocontin two nocte. He has much improved until mid-January when I gave him a short course of prednisolone. Now he is still SOB, BP 180/100. Chest clear. I have added Becotide inhaler tds and would be grateful for your advice.

Response: 'Thank you for referring this life-long non-smoker. He enjoyed very good health till retirement. Over the last few months he has experienced episodes of dyspnoea, coughing, heaviness of chest, orthopnoea and paroxysmal nocturnal dyspnoea. His ankles are swollen. There is very little sputum.

On examination he looked well. He became breathless on undressing. BP was 190/105. JVP was raised and he has clinically enlarged left ventricle. There was bilateral basal rhonchi and crepitations. FEV_1 1.7 l, FVC 3.7 l, PEFR 480 l/min. Chest X-ray showed cardiomegaly. ECG showed left heart strain and early ischaemia.

I believe that he has late-onset asthma but also left heart failure secondary to hypertension. I have maintained him on Becotide, Intal, prednisone and added Navidrex K two daily and will see him again shortly'.

Progress: Two months later, he was much better – no longer breathless at night and lost 3 kg in weight – having had good diuresis. Chest X-ray showed decrease in heart size and BP was 170/90. Intal and Becotide caused irritation and dysphonia and he stopped using these without any worsening of asthma. Patient maintained on steroids, diuretics and salbutamol for the next five years with good blood pressure control and PEFR often 600 l/min.

In 1986, marked steroid muscle wasting was noted. Recommencing inhaled treatment (including Atrovent and Duovent) produced no reduction in steroid dose (10–15 mg daily), adrenal suppression confirmed (Synacthen test). A short course of anabolic steroids given with effect. He remained well.

Comment: This patient again demonstrates that late-onset asthma is often intrinsic, unpredictable and steroid-dependent. He also shows that it is often difficult to distinguish between bronchial asthma and left heart insufficiency ('cardiac asthma'). Of course, β-blockers of all types should be avoided in asthmatics with hypertension or ischaemic heart disease. Dysphonia can be a troublesome symptom in patients who regularly take steroid medication via the inhaled route.

REPORT NUMBER 6

A 37-year-old housewife was referred in March 1985.

GPs letter: 'Thank you very much for seeing this lady who has, until recently, been under the care of Dr —— at —— Hospital. She had aspergillosis diagnosed six years ago and is still having three-monthly follow-ups.

She asked me if she can be transferred to you and I would be grateful for your advice. Thank you very much.'

Response: 'Many thanks indeed for asking me to see this pleasant non-smoking lady whose brother has asthma and hay fever.

She has had hay fever and eczema and also intermittent wheezing of asthma. She was told some years ago that she also had aspergillosis and had collapse of parts of her left lung because of sputum plugs.

She has only recently finished a course of prednisolone, and in spite of this she has cough, wheeze and distress. She feels tired.

Her chest revealed polyphonic wheezes but no evidence of collapse. She has patches of eczema and evidence of rhinitis.

FEV_1 1.2 l, PEFR 350 l/min. Urine showed trace of protein only. Chest X-ray shows patchy pneumonitis consistent with aspergillosis. There was marked eosinophilia (blood) but ESR was 17.

I have told her that the best way of preventing long-term lung damage from aspergillosis is to treat the asthma as well, and in view of her poor lung function tests, I think she will need to maintain on steroids (maintenance) for the next six months. I do not feel that repeat of allergy tests would help as she reacted positively to most allergens. So I have kept her on prednisolone 5 mg per day and will see her again shortly.'

Progress: She remained well for the subsequent six months but needed prednisolone 10–15 mg daily. Triamcinolone (Kenalog) injections, although successful in reducing prednisone dose to 2.5 mg daily, produced dysfunctional uterine bleeding and was not given again. In 1986 she had collapse of right upper lobe – bronchoscopy showed obstruction due to thick aspergillus plugs. In January 1987 in an effort to stop 'steroids', she had 'hypnosis' and remained off prednisolone till May 1987 with progressive deterioration in lung function tests and further collapse of right upper lobe. She has now recommenced steroids and is well.

Comment: Pulmonary aspergillosis and asthma occurring in young individuals can be very disabling and without regular steroids and supervision may result in classic severe disability with the complications of fibrosis and cor pulmonale. Respiratory failure is likely.

REPORT NUMBER 7

A 26-year-old man was admitted to hospital urgently.

GPs letter: 'Thank you for admitting this young man whose asthma – normally well controlled – has become worse over the past two days in spite of antibiotics, Phyllocontin and changing Becotide to Becloforte'.

Discharge letter: 'This 26-year-old non-smoking factory worker was known to have had asthma since childhood. He has also had eczema, hay fever, nasal polyps and ?milk allergy. There is a strong family history of some of these disorders. He has never been admitted to hospital as an emergency nor has he attended any hospital clinics. We gather that allergy tests in his childhood showed him to be allergic to most things and he had a course of 'densensitization' injections between the age of 5–9 years.

He has had upper respiratory tract infection over the past week which has caused worsening of his asthma. He has not been able to work because of persistent cough, wheeze and tightness. He had been unable to sleep for two days because of the cough and dyspnoea.

He was very distressed and frightened; pulse was 112/min, paradox >20 mm. He had mild fever. Respiratory rate >30/min. Chest was 'silent'. PEFR was 85 l/min, i.e. 15% of predicted normal level. pO_2 was 8.2 kPa and pCO_2 was 5.9 kPa.

He was nursed on the ITU with 35% oxygen, intravenous hydrocortisone, nebulized salbutamol and ipratropium. Becloforte was stopped *pro-tem*. Intravenous aminophylline was not given because of risk of theophylline toxicity as he had received slow-release theophylline from you. Hydration was maintained, antibiotics course was continued.

He improved quickly, pO_2 rising to 13.2 kPa and pCO_2 4.7 kPa. PEFR rose eventually to 540 l/min. There was no early morning 'dip' on the PEFR reading and he was discharged on the following:

EC prednisolone 5 mg tds to eventually stop in 3 weeks;

Becloforte 2 puffs bd to change to Becotide if appropriate; and

Ipratropium bromide (Atrovent) 2 puffs bd and salbutamol as necessary

We recommend that a course of steroids (10 days) be left with the patient and he would take these in the event of further acute exacerbation. A peak flow meter has been loaned to him and he has been asked to maintain PEFR >450 l/min.

Comment (1) This patient had never before – even during acute exacerbations when he had taken long periods off work – received steroids, (2) there was no previous record of PEFR, and (3) the patient's asthma state on admission to hospital had become critical.

REPORT NUMBER 8

A 16-year-old schoolboy was referred in July 1986.

GPs letter: 'This young lad has been previously very fit and healthy. There is no family history of asthma but he has attended here regularly with symptoms of breathlessness suggesting bronchospasm. No amount of bronchodilator therapy would help – steroids were also useless. Would you kindly advise on further management.'

Response: 'Many thanks for asking me to see this sensitive, intelligent young lad who has as yet not smoked. His symptoms are of "panicky" breathlessness – occurring at any time and described as "unable to fill my lungs – air would not go in". Inhalers worsen the situation. He has used one salbutamol inhaler over a few days, he is otherwise well.

He looked withdrawn and worried. On being asked to take deep breaths, he started to hyperventilate. Chest was clear. FEV_1 3.0 l, FVC 4.2 l and PEFR 520 l/min, chest X-ray normal. pO_2 11.7 kPa, pCO_2 3.2 kPa. Allergy tests (prick) were negative.

I think this boy has anxiety induced dyspnoea – the so-called dysproportionate dyspnoea. I have obtained from him the reason why he is in this state and explained the remedy. All therapy can be stopped.'

Comment: The reason for this patient's symptoms of breathlessness was emotional. The family had decided to move to another country – this the boy was very apprehensive about because of change of school and the fact that he was leaving friends behind. He had not related his anxieties to his parents and was relieved to talk about them in front of his mother. The family decided eventually to delay the move with dramatic improvement in the boy's symptoms and outlook.

REPORT NUMBER 9

A 60-year-old woman was referred in October 1985.

GPs letter: 'This lady has been asthmatic over the course of the last year which unfortunately has not improved very much and her peak flow is only 200 l/min.

At the present moment she is using Becotide and Ventolin, but I tried Provent and also in July gave an injection of Kenalog. This, unfortunately, did not make any difference and I am not sure if anything further can be done to improve her breathing but I would appreciate your views.'

Response: 'Many thanks indeed for asking me to see this lady who has had a previous problem with her right arm and this has been localized to an ulnar nerve involvement. She has a lot of wasting.

She gave me a 12 month history of being unwell with increasing breathlessness, some weight loss, anorexia and a few episodes of haemoptysis. Her son has asthma and the wheezing she had could easily be mistaken for this condition developing in her.

Looking at her I thought the physical signs were more of left upper lobe collapse. She also had some facial weakness and I hope this does not indicate any central nervous system disturbance.

FEV_1 1.2 l, FVC 1.6 l and PEFR 180 l/min.

I have looked at her previous X-rays in May and July 1985. These show a straight left heart border. Her repeat film now unfortunately confirms the clinical impression of the left upper lobe collapse.

She is a heavy smoker (over 30 cigarettes a day) and I think there can be very little doubt that she has a slow-growing squamous cell cancer of the left upper lobe. This may still be operable if we can exclude metastasis, although her lung function tests are extremely poor. However, she needs detailed assessment, especially with regards to her relatively young age and I am taking her into hospital to do this, and will let you have more information shortly.'

Progress: Diagnosis of inoperable squamous cell carcinoma of left lower lobe was confirmed on bronchoscopy. She has received a palliative course of radiotherapy and in June 1987 remains well with no obvious evidence of metastases. She is not taking any therapy.

Comments:

(1) A straight left heart border in a smoker with persistent respiratory symptoms may mean early collapse of left lower lobe and needs further assessment including bronchoscopy.

(2) Upper and lower airways obstruction secondary to tumour or other foreign bodies may mimic asthma. Flow volume loops (curves) may help distinguish upper from lower airway narrowing.

(3) Diagnosis of asthma in heavy smoking patients of middle age should always be under close scrutiny and these patients need regular review by the doctor.

REPORT NUMBER 10

A 9-year-old girl was referred in October 1983.

GPs letter: 'Thank you so much for seeing this 9-year-old girl who has been troubled with some wheezing over the past five years or so. She has a younger brother with a similar complaint. Five years or so ago her bronchospasm started to appear, usually associated with an upper respiratory tract infection and in recent months we have been using Intal routinely to prevent bronchospasm. She had pharyngitis which produced marked bronchospasm and she fortunately recovered taking antibiotics and a Duovent inhaler. I would greatly value your opinion on any further management that might reduce this girl's attacks of bronchospasm.'

Response: 'Many thanks indeed for asking me to see this very pleasant and intelligent girl who has, over the years, been struggling with wheeze, cough and nocturnal misery. Her performance at school and on exercise is now becoming of great concern.

She looked well but became very wheezy on undressing. There were polyphonic wheezes in both lung fields. FEV_1 0.4 l, FVC 0.8 l, PEFR 120 l/min. Chest X-ray was normal. Allergy tests were negative.

This is severe intrinsic asthma. I have suggested that she uses Becotide inhaler twice a day with her Duovent also twice a day and salbutamol as required. I have given her an injection of triamcinolone 40 mg im and will see her again.'

Progress: When seen in December 1983, she had abandoned Nuelin, aminophylline, Intal and Duovent and only took Becotide and salbutamol twice a day. PEFR had risen to 240 l/min, she had no time off school and was very active – swimming for the first time.

Over the subsequent two years, she needed a few depo-steroid injections but remained very well. In 1986, no depo-steroid was necessary and she used salbutamol and Becotide very infrequently. On assessment in May 1987, PEFR was 360 l/min and she was discharged back to the general practitioner.

REPORT NUMBER 11

A 34-year-old civil servant was referred in January 1985.

GPs letter: 'This young non-smoking man has been greatly troubled by persistent cough, wheeze and tightness for the past year. I have used all the bronchodilating medication known to me, including steroids, but no good. Would you kindly help!

Response: 'Many thanks for asking me to see this man who had mild eczema and asthma in his early childhood. There is family history of allergy. He, as you say, has had no problems in the 'teens but over the past 18 months noticed progressive disability due to cough (dry) – worse at night – and wheeze and tightness on exercise. He had to give up jogging. His general health otherwise is satisfactory.

Examination was unremarkable. Chest X-ray was normal. FEV_1 1.7 l, FVC 3.4 l and PEFR 270 l/min. Allergy tests were negative.

He presents an interesting problem. About the time his asthma returned, upon his wife's suggestion, he took up a "hobby" of photography, developing films in the "boxroom" in the house. This is poorly ventilated. I think this may be contributing or causing his asthma. He says when on holidays – away from the "hobby" at which he has become very successful – he feels "fine", needing no inhalers or other medication. I have therefore suggested to him the probable connection. It came as a surprise to him. It would be interesting to see what happens when he abandons his "hobby" – reluctantly!'

Progress: On discussion with his wife, the couple initially locked the room where 'developing' took place, with the result that there was complete relief from asthma.

Comment: This has to be regarded as a form of 'occupational' asthma, caused probably by a silver-based solution used in developing in a confined space. It is necessary when taking history from an asthmatic to include the following:

(1) pets;

(2) materials used in bedding;
(3) soap powder;
(4) occupation; and
(5) hobbies.

REPORT NUMBER 12

A 47-year-old pharmacist was referred in July 1985.

GPs letter: 'I would be grateful is you could see this lady whose episodic wheezing and breathlessness over the past few months has not responded to any bronchodilator or steroid therapy. She is very disabled and now has chest pain.'

Response: 'Many thanks for sending this non-smoking woman. There is no previous history of allergy syndrome and she denies family history of these problems.

Over the past few months, she has had periods of 'tight' breathlessness, dizziness and pleuritic chest pain. These symptoms have at times occurred at night and are particularly frequent before her menstrual periods.

Examination revealed generally a well lady with regular pulse and blood pressure. She had some coarse crackles and probable pleural rub at the left base. There were no significant varicose veins but calves were tender on palpation.

FEV_1 was 2.1 l, FVC 3.0 l, PEFR 480 l/min. Chest X-ray showed slightly elevated left diaphragm. Electrocardiograph was normal.

I feel that this is not bronchial asthma but more likely to be recurrent pulmonary emboli. I have admitted her to hospital.'

Progress: Her bronchodilator therapy was stopped and she was given heparin. Lung scan (V/Q) confirmed bilateral pulmonary emboli, left leg venogram showed extensive deep vein thrombosis.

She remained very well on warfarin; this was stopped after six months. She remains well.

REPORT NUMBER 13

A 58-year-old was referred in January 1987.

GPs letter: 'This patient wishes to have some further advice for her allergic problems. She has a long history of asthma and uses a Ventolin inhaler at least once a day. Her eyes are sore or dry on wakening and also wet with some irritation. She has otitis externa and eczema of the pinna and tells me that her nose is often blocked. I am grateful to you for seeing her and for your help with further investigations.'

Response: 'Many thanks indeed for your letter and for asking me to see this member of our staff here. She has been virtually a non-smoker, there is no family history of allergy. She developed hay fever at the age of nine but does not have any symptoms now. She then had asthma, and in the 1960s developed eczema. Allergy tests in her teens were positive to feathers, house dust, cat fur and dog hair. She had a course of desensitizing injections. Her symptoms now are of rhinitis, conjunctivitis, wheezy breathlessness and candida-like discharge with mucus passed in her stools. She feels generally tired.

Examination was satisfactory. Chest X-ray was normal. FEV_1 was 2.0 l, FVC 2.8 l and PEFR 445 l/min.

I suspect the asthmatic component is not very significant at the moment and her main problem is secondary to nasal allergy. She has had an operation for a deviated nasal septum in the past. I have asked for X-rays of her sinuses, allergy tests (including RAST) and will see her again shortly for further advice.'

Results: Sinuses: 'There is extensive polypoid mucosal thickening in the right antrum and there is also some thickening present on the lateral wall of the left antrum. No other abnormality.'

Serum total IgE >400 U/ml (normal less than 140 U/ml).
Allergy tests (prick):

House dust 7 mm

House dust mite 10 mm
Grass pollen 12 mm
Rye 14 mm
Dog 8 mm
Cat 8 mm

Aspergillus, yeast, chocolate, milk, egg, cheese – negative. Specific IgE (RAST): moderate to high significant result in house dust mite, mixed grass pollen, trees and weeds.

Progress: Patient was advised to use Beconase nasal spray twice a day and Beclomethasone inhaler 2 puffs also twice a day. When seen four weeks later there was very significant improvement in rhinitis, headaches, wheezing and 'mucus' discharge. She continues on this regime. Desensitization would be considered in future as second line of management.

Comment: It is possible in certain very 'allergic' individuals to have migraine, lack of concentration and 'mucus' in the stools. This patient had all these three and improving her nasal problems resulted in relief from the other symptoms.

REPORT NUMBER 14

A 49-year-old postal worker was referred in November 1986.

GPs letter: 'Thank you for seeing this man who has suffered from intermittent asthma since childhood. He came to see me in September with a dry cough and wheeze. This responded moderately well with salbutamol spandets and when I saw him again his peak flow with 460 with only a localized wheeze in the upper zones suggestive of bronchitis. However, courses of Septrin and Augmentin did not help his breathlessness by early October. I started him on reducing courses of prednisone and Ventolin inhaler whilst awaiting a chest X-ray. The latter was normal and he felt much better when the prednisone was finished. Unfortunately his asthma has relapsed and he is too breathless to work. This has been despite starting Slo-phyllin and Becotide. He has now lost a lot of income because of asthma, and has requested referral. I have had him back on steroids reducing to a maintenance dose of one daily and have increased Slo-phyllin to two tablets bd whilst continuing the Ventolin inhaler in the hope that we may be able to get him back to his job. I would appreciate your opinion.'

Response: 'Many thanks indeed for asking me to see this relatively young man who is a non-smoker. He admits to persistant asthma for three months. Physical examination revealed disabling severe bronchospasm. He had tachycardia, significant paradox and PEFR 110 l/min. He was not able to record FEV_1 and FVC. Chest X-ray was normal. Allergy tests showed moderate reaction to house-dust and 'mite' only.

He therefore has severe acute asthma. I have admitted him to hospital.'

Progress: He was given parenteral steroids (hydrocortisone) and nebulized salbutamol, ipratropium (Atrovent) and Becotide and Phyllocontin continued. PEFR rose gradually and he still manifested 'early morning dip' for a few days. Over the subsequent week improvement continued and he achieved a PEFR >500 l/min with no 'dips' and normal arterial blood gases (pO_2/pCO_2). He was discharged using salbutamol and Atrovent via a home nebulizer, Becotide inhaler twice a day and reducing prednisone over the next month and stopping it altogether. On review a few months later he had not lost any time off work, not needed any prednisone and took other treatment regularly. PEFR averaged 525 l/min.

Comment: This patient demonstrates very well the benefits of home nebulized treatment.

MULTIPLE CHOICE QUESTIONS

(1) The original derivation of the word asthma from Greek literature meant:
  (a) Difficulty in breathing
  (b) I suffocate
  (c) Prolonged coughing
  (d) Respiratory distress
  (e) Wheezing at night

(2) Incidence of asthma in general population:
  (a) 20%
  (b) 3%
  (c) 7%
  (d) 2%
  (e) 1%

(3) Number of deaths (annual) in UK attributed to asthma:
  (a) 50 000
  (b) 15 000
  (c) 1500
  (d) 500
  (e) 100

(4) Estimated asthmatics in USA:
   (a) 100 000
   (b) 500 000
   (c) 2 million
   (d) 3 million
   (e) 6–8 million

(5) 'Soap-powder asthma' – which of the following are implicated:
   (a) Dust particle size
   (b) Direct toxicity
   (c) Sensitization to enzyme of *Bacillus subtilis*
   (d) Incidence rising
   (e) Effects irreversible

(6) Which of the following groups of drugs are best avoided in any asthmatic:
   (a) Aspirin
   (b) Ephedrine
   (c) β-Blockers
   (d) Non-steroidal anti-inflammatory drugs (NSAIDs)
   (e) Opiates

(7) Which of the following are unusual in asthma:
   (a) Finger clubbing
   (b) Persistent basal inspiratory crackles in both lungs
   (c) Stridor
   (d) 'Silent' chest in acute severe state
   (e) Confusion and aggression in acute asthma

(8) The following are true statements:
   (a) We do not know the cause of an asthma attack
   (b) Genetic aspect very significant
   (c) Extrinsic asthma less common in boys
   (d) Aspirin particularly hazardous in intrinsic asthmatic with nasal polyps
   (e) 'Atopic' deaths common in the elderly

(9) The mast cell – which of the following are true statements:
   (a) Forms the largest percentage of airway cells
   (b) Direct relationship between the number of cells and airway hypersensitivity
   (c) Responsible for secretion of prostaglandin
   (d) Not responsible for secretion of leukotrienes
   (e) Less significant in intrinsic asthma

(10) About asthma deaths – which of the following are true:
- (a) Peaked in mid-1960s
- (b) Female death rate much higher
- (c) Wider use of home nebulizer may contribute
- (d) Most at risk at night
- (e) Geographical variation (world-wide)

(11) Recorded 'dips' in PEFR will occur:
- (a) In an asymptomatic patient
- (b) Mid-morning
- (c) On exercise
- (d) On exposure to smoke
- (e) On exposure to cold air

(12) Airway hyper-responsiveness occurs in:
- (a) Exposure to epoxyresins
- (b) RSV infection
- (c) Bacterial pneumonia
- (d) Stress
- (e) General anaesthesia

(13) Histopathology of sputum in asthma would commonly reveal:
- (a) *Aspergillus* species
- (b) Eosinophils
- (c) Curschmann's spirals
- (d) Metaplastic cells
- (e) Charcot–Leyden crystals

(14) Asthmatic syndromes occur in:
- (a) Polyarteritis nodosa
- (b) Polymyalgia rheumatica
- (c) Allergic alveolitis (farmer's lung)
- (d) Fibrosing alveolitis (cryptogenic fibrosis)
- (e) Psittacosis

(15) Problems of inhaled steroids include:
- (a) Severe adrenal suppression
- (b) Oral candidiasis
- (c) Irreversible vocal cord paresis
- (d) Tracheal ulceration
- (e) Hypersensitivity

(16) Which of the following groups of people are best thought to educate patients in technique of inhalation:
(a) Doctors
(b) Nurses
(c) Physiotherapist
(d) Relatives
(e) Medical students

(17) Which of the following are available in solutions for the nebulizer:
(a) Ipratropium bromide (Atrovent)
(b) Beclomethasone
(c) Disodium cromoglycate (Intal)
(d) Terbutaline
(e) Fenoterol (Berotec)

(18) When parenteral (iv) theophylline used in acute severe asthma:
(a) Previous intake of slow-release preparations of theophylline should exclude this group from such treatment
(b) Avoided in pregnant patient
(c) Used with care in heavy smokers
(d) Blood levels not necessary
(e) Can be cardiotoxic

(19) Sodium cromoglycate – which of the following is true:
(a) Very effective in intrinsic asthma
(b) Has effect on influx of magnesium ions
(c) Is safe
(d) Treatment should be on a regular basis
(e) Was introduced in 1947

(20) Nedocromil sodium (Tilade) – which of the following is true:
(a) Much more effective than regular doses of inhaled steroids
(b) Introduced in 1982 in UK
(c) It has an added anti-inflammatory property
(d) Should not be used with β_2-agonists
(e) Has a potent effect on histamine release

(21) Triamcinolone (Kenalog) in asthma – which of the following is true:
(a) A very effective alternative to oral steroids
(b) Particularly useful in intrinsic asthma
(c) Side-effects rare when used regularly
(d) Bruising is reversible
(e) Cheaper when compared with other conventional forms of treatment

(22) Exercise–induced asthma – which of the following is true:
- (a) Uncommon as a precipitating factor
- (b) Wheezing occurs immediately on commencing exercise
- (c) Beta-agonists preferred
- (d) Ipratroprium bromide (Atrovent) very effective in certain groups
- (e) Poor prognosis

(23) Acute severe asthma – which of the following is true:
- (a) Tachycardia >110/min
- (b) Peak flow rate <25% predicted
- (c) Acute right heart strain may occur
- (d) Pneumothorax possible
- (e) Sedatives justified in aggressive, confused patient

(24) A pregnant asthmatic – which of the following is true:
- (a) Should always be referred to a specialist for asthma management
- (b) Condition will invariably worsen
- (c) Theophyllines produce no teratogenicity
- (d) Steroids must be avoided
- (e) Asthma recurs with subsequent pregnancies

(25) The following hold their place for future research in asthma:
- (a) Immunotherapy
- (b) Beta-agonist pro-drugs
- (c) Calcium antagonists
- (d) Anti-thromboxane drugs
- (e) Hypnosis

ANSWERS

(1) (a) × (b) √ (c) × (d) × (e) ×
(2) (a) × (b) × (c) √ (d) × (e) ×
(3) (a) × (b) × (c) √ (d) × (e) ×
(4) (a) × (b) × (c) × (d) × (e) √
(5) (a) × (b) × (c) √ (d) √ (e) ×
(6) (a) √ (b) × (c) √ (d) × (e) √
(7) (a) √ (b) √ (c) √ (d) × (e) ×
(8) (a) √ (b) × (c) × (d) √ (e) ×
(9) (a) × (b) × (c) √ (d) × (e) ×
(10) (a) √ (b) × (c) × (d) √ (e) √
(11) (a) √ (b) × (c) √ (d) √ (e) √
(12) (a) √ (b) √ (c) √ (d) √ (e) ×
(13) (a) × (b) √ (c) √ (d) × (e) √
(14) (a) √ (b) × (c) √ (d) × (e) ×
(15) (a) × (b) √ (c) × (d) √ (e) ×
(16) (a) × (b) × (c) √ (d) √ (e) ×
(17) (a) √ (b) √ (c) √ (d) √ (e) √
(18) (a) √ (b) × (c) √ (d) × (e) ×
(19) (a) × (b) × (c) √ (d) √ (e) ×
(20) (a) × (b) × (c) √ (d) × (e) ×
(21) (a) √ (b) √ (c) × (d) √ (e) √
(22) (a) × (b) × (c) √ (d) √ (e) ×
(23) (a) √ (b) √ (c) √ (d) √ (e) ×
(24) (a) × (b) × (c) √ (d) × (e) ×
(25) (a) √ (b) √ (c) × (d) √ (e) ×

INDEX

macrophage

Inhibitors:
Trental

mast cell (Atopics)

leukotriene

prostaglandin — Indocin OK4-046 — Virus

thromboxane — Indocin OK4-046 — Virus

eosinophils - eos in blood (Atopics ?)

platelets - (Atopic ?)

neutrophils